PENGUIN BOOKS

QUEER AND LOATHING

David B. Feinberg, a graduate of M.I.T., is the author of the novels *Eighty-Six* Literary Award for Gay Men's Fiction and America Association Gay/Lesbian Book Award for Fiction) and *Spon* Stories, articles, and reviews by him appeared in *The New York Times Book Review*, *The Advocate*, *Details*, *Outweek*, *Tribe*, *NYQ*, *QW*, *Out*, *The Body Positive*, *Gay Community News*, *Art & Understanding*, *The James White Review*, *Diseased Pariah News*, *Poz*, and both *Men on Men 2: Best New Gay Fiction* and *Men on Men 4*. Mr. Feinberg died in New York City of AIDS-related complications on November 2, 1994; he was thirty-seven.

• •

Praise for *Queer and Loathing*

"David Feinberg delineates and populates the vast, maddening, fascinating universe of being HIV-positive in our time better and more fully than virtually every AIDS novel I've read. His feline ability to twist and turn into the best possible position when he lands after a fall of twenty-five floors is just one element of what makes the book such a wonderful read. His sense of optimism despite the crushingly depressing nature of the material is strangely joyous. And his pleasure in writing for you and to you, despite the cost to himself, is a delight."
  —Felice Picano, *Lambda Book Report*

"Horrifyingly funny, profoundly human, and truthful to the point of murder. It's not just a good book, it's an important book. I believe it will endure."
  —Michael Cunningham, author of *Flesh and Blood*

"*Queer and Loathing* displays the combination of razor-sharp black humor and frustration with moral injustice that worked to great effect in Feinberg's novels. It is a moving testament to the author's indomitable spirit."
  —Michael Lowenthal, *Boston Phoenix Literary Supplement*

"This wickedly funny, rollercoaster ride of a book is an important addition to the library of anyone concerned with the future of humankind."
  —*In the Life*

Queer and Loathing

RANTS AND RAVES
OF A RAGING
AIDS CLONE

David B. Feinberg

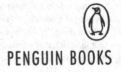

PENGUIN BOOKS

PENGUIN BOOKS
Published by the Penguin Group
Penguin Books USA Inc., 375 Hudson Street, New York, New York 10014, U.S.A.
Penguin Books Ltd, 27 Wrights Lane, London W8 5TZ, England
Penguin Books Australia Ltd, Ringwood, Victoria, Australia
Penguin Books Canada Ltd, 10 Alcorn Avenue, Toronto, Ontario, Canada M4V 3B2
Penguin Books (N.Z.) Ltd, 182–190 Wairau Road, Auckland 10, New Zealand

Penguin Books Ltd, Registered Offices: Harmondsworth, Middlesex, England

First published in the United States of America by Viking Penguin,
a division of Penguin Books USA Inc., 1994
This edition with a preface by Tony Kushner published in Penguin Books 1995

"Queer and Loathing at the FDA: Revolt of the Perverts" first appeared in *Tribe*;
"Etiquette for the HIV-Antibody-Positive in *Body Positive*; "Notes from the Front
Lines: Writing about AIDS," "Direct Mail from Hell," and "April Fools" (as "Getting
AIDS Absurd") in *NYQ*; "Tales from the Front" and "The AIDS Clone vs. the New
Clone" in *Diseased Pariah News*; "Sex Tips for Boys" and "Cocktails from Hell" in
QW; "AIDS and Humor" (as "Is Humor an Acceptable Way to Deal with AIDS?")
in *The Advocate*; "100 Ways You Can Fight the AIDS Crisis" in LIFEbeat concert
fund-raiser program; "Waiting for the End of the World" in *Art & Understanding*;
"Memorials from Hell" in *Gay Community News*; "A Season in Hell" (as "HIV +
Me") in *Details*; and "Death Be Not Proud" (as "Urn Your Keep") in *Out*.

THE LIBRARY OF CONGRESS HAS CATALOGUED THE HARDCOVER AS FOLLOWS:
Feinberg, David B.
Queer and loathing: rants and raves of a raging AIDS clone/David B. Feinberg.
p.   cm.
ISBN 0-670-85766-1 (hc.)
ISBN 0 14 02.4080 2 (pbk.)
1. AIDS (Disease)   2. HIV infections.   3. Gay Men—United States.   I. Title.
RA644.A25F45 1994
362.1'969792—dc20   94–5074

Printed in the United States of America
Set in Bembo
Designed by Brian Mulligan

In Memory of Bob Rafsky

Thanks to my friends
Wayne Allen Kawadler,
Jan Carl Park,
and John Palmer Weir, Jr.

Contents

Preface

The AIDS epidemic came along and ripped open reality, ir-
reparably, irretrievably. All expectations have been violated, all
guarantees of life-as-usual are declared null-and-void. Through
this great gaping tear, through this wound, much pain, un-
countable losses, and insuperable grief have issued; and also
much rage, much courage, much hard-won intelligence, and
even some wisdom. David Feinberg would have been an important writer even if we'd all been spared the last ten years. His encounter with what we haven't been spared—and we haven't
been spared much—has produced work that holds its audience
excruciatingly on the razor's edge between comedy and horror.
Feinberg makes you laugh from precisely the place inside of you
where laughter really hurts. There's a terrible, cumulative effect
in reading these essays: coruscating, moving, outraged and outrageous, they chronicle the travels and travails of our own Jere-
miah, or better yet, our Amos, the soul-baring, self-exposing,
unsparing moralist—a prophetic voice at any rate, with the
added grace note of a blistering sense of humor, without which
life in this charnel-house of a century is inconceivable.

Feinberg's bitter, finely titrated bile, his refusal to despair and his scrupulous recording of despair's many temptations, his witty observant eye, his compassion and his morality and his take-no-prisoners invective: these are some of the qualities that make him unique, and uniquely important, among the chroniclers of our plague. This is writing that refuses to offer any palliatives, that seeks to intensify what is already unbearable. This is the harshest, and most brave, and most necessary kind of art.

—Tony Kushner
March 1995

Introduction

I've been straddling the line between fiction and fact for quite some time now. In *Eighty-Sixed* and *Spontaneous Combustion* I filtered my experiences through a fictional persona, B. J. Rosenthal. This mask allowed me to selectively reshape my past. Yet I found that the more I wrote, the fewer alterations of fact I made. I was moving closer toward the truth.

Now it's time to come clean. *Queer and Loathing* is a collection of essays on AIDS. Somewhat less than half have been previously published, in somewhat different form; the opening pages of these indicate the place and date of original publication. I added endnotes to place them in context. I also added endnotes to some of the previously unpublished pieces.

I've always attempted to tell the truth in my writing. I've tried to capture what is to me a painfully obvious reality that is rarely written about: what it is like for a gay man to live in the epicenter of the AIDS epidemic; what it is like to be HIV-positive in the nineties; what it is like to outlive one therapist, two dentists, two doctors, and one gastroenterologist. At times I'm shocked when I feel that no one else is documenting this personal history without transmuting it to some metaphoric plane.

There is no literal truth, of course. Truth is a philosophical invention one can only approach. All writing is lies. Good writing is lies skillfully told.

Some minor details have been altered in *Queer and Loathing*. Some names have been changed. As I dance at the border of fiction and fact, this is as close to the truth as I can get.

Part
One

Queer
and
Loathing

Queer and Loathing at the FDA: Revolt of the Perverts

Introduction

I'm writing this down during the twilight of Western civilization as we know it. My editor has chained me to my personal computer. Periodically I doze off, and the keyboard, equipped with a simple mechanism, wakes me with a jolt of electroshock. The deadline is long past. The powers that be are feeding me a combination of legal and illegal stimulants, further deranging my normally irrational powers of cogitation. I sit here exhausted, suffering from a plethora of imaginary maladies and ailments, recalling October 11, 1988, the day some fifteen hundred fags and dykes and AIDS activists and sympathizers *seized control of the Food and Drug Administration*.

There's only one way to tell my story: eighties gonzo journalism. Let me take this opportunity to inform you from the start that I have complete and total contempt for you, my dear reader. I want to bite the hand that feeds me, and *surgical gloves won't save you*. I've read the surveys in *Rolling Stone* and I know that 95 percent of you thirtysomething motherfuckers wouldn't mind having

Originally appeared in Tribe, *Vol. 1, No. 1, Winter 1989.*

an individual of the Negro persuasion move next door, but 58 percent don't want a fag to date your brother. *I've got your number.* I know that most of you dungbrains are just chock-full of compassion for people with AIDS as long as they aren't queers or junkies. Pity the poor, innocent babies and the unsuspecting wives of bisexuals, but ignore the growing mounds of corpses right in front of your eyes.

I'm sick and tired of all of this talk about innocent victims. *I plead guilty.* I'm guilty of crimes against nature. I have done truly abominable things according to Leviticus, Deuteronomy, and the collected works of Jackie Collins. I'm the Jew that poisoned the wells; I'm the pinko that passed the atomic spy plans to the Russkies; I'm the Toon that framed Roger Rabbit. I'm the one *my own parents* warned me against.

I'm sitting here at my desk, tanked up on Heineken, amphetamines, and sugar at the four A.M. of your soul. I plead guilty with the Twinkie defense.

Yes, I have seduced fifteen-year-old boys on anti-nuke marches, I have blasphemed Christ Our Lord repeatedly, I have been a card-carrying member of the ACLU for longer than I care to remember, I have had sex in places both public and private that would shock most of Middle America, I have spilled my seed while watching videos that cannot be sold in certain states south of the Mason-Dixon Line. I have done all of the things you expected me to do, and much, much more.

Let me warn you: I am a pathological liar. Not a single word of this is true. What follows is an amalgamation of rumors, innuendos, and gross exaggerations; hyperbole, paranoia, and third-stage dementia. *This is how far you have driven me.* Everything is subjective. Names and faces have been changed due to incontinence of the memory and a desire to cloud the past with a haze of hydrophobic rage. At this point facts are immaterial. To quote Lily Tomlin, reality is for people who can't cope with drugs.

Sex and Drugs and Rock and Roll

To make it simple for you pinheads out there, think of me as a junkie. Like any other addict, I'm prepared to slice your bleeding liberal heart into ribbons *in order to get my drugs.* These are some of the drugs that I need: aerosol pentamidine, acyclovir, azidothymidine, AL721, dextran sulfate, naltrexone, Antabuse, foscarnet, Imuthiol, CD4, and Ampligen. It's *Valley of the Dolls in the Valley of the Shadow of Death.* There are one hundred thirty drugs out there that show promise against the HIV virus, and at this writing the FDA has approved two. I have no intention of flying to France for Imuthiol, or Mexico for ribavirin. *I want my drugs—and I want them now.* The way things are going, I might not even be allowed to leave the country when the estimated one and a half million infected with the virus are quarantined to the United States. The way things are going, some crazed right-wing lunatic like Representative William Dannemeyer could try to turn Wyoming into a concentration camp.

How, you may ask, did I end up in this virulent state of desperation? Was it *sex and drugs and rock and roll?* Did I sleep with an IV-drug abuser at Heartbreak Hotel in Loisaida, after sharing works with him? Am I an angry fetus, about to be born with a habit and a life expectancy of *less than zero?* Did I get the wrong transfusion five years ago? Or am I just sick and tired of watching my friends die?

It's none of your goddamned business.

You'd probably be surprised to hear it, but at heart I'm a Puritan. I'm L-seven, square. I don't drink, smoke, or do recreational drugs. *I don't like to have fun.* So what the fuck am I doing demonstrating for drugs? Why am I mainlining AIDS activism in the form of ACT UP? The answer is quite simple. *I want to stay alive.* It's the Basic Survival Instinct. I don't want to have to wait eight to ten years to have the drugs of choice approved by the Food and Drug Administration so some lackey at a cemetery can infuse my rotting corpse with them.

Why I Went to Demonstrate at the FDA

I can't argue *anything*. Throw me into a closet for three weeks and I'll become a Symbionese Liberation Terrorist, but only if you rape me. It's the Stockholm Syndrome all over. Arguments are so—so—*dissentive*. What I mean to say is that I am completely inarticulate in person. Shove a mike into my face and I'm more likely to fellate it than spout revolutionary drivel. My problem is that I can empathize with *anyone;* I look at *every* side of an argument, weigh *all* of the pros and cons, and then come to a decision. Just about anyone can sway me with the right techniques: charm, wit, style, grace, intelligence, physical attractiveness, penis size, oral technique, or large unmarked bills.

So once I've decided something, I stick with it. Even though I may not be able to recall the individual factors, even though my reasons are no longer clear, I remain steadfast. I am only articulate with explanations on paper.

I am going to have to burden you with some facts. I'm sorry; I don't want to tax your minuscule cranial capacities. Don't worry, *there won't be a quiz*. I'll spoon-feed everything to you.

The Food and Drug Administration is set up to regulate and approve drugs that are both safe and effective. We don't want any more babies born with flippers; scratch thalidomide, a sedative prescribed in Europe during the late fifties that caused severe birth defects. We don't want any more sideshow barkers shilling snake oil; we don't want people to go to Mexico for ineffective drugs like apricot pits to arrest cancer, while ignoring other useful therapies. But at this point in time, there's AZT for AIDS, and that's it. About half of the people with AIDS either can't take AZT because it's too toxic or experience no improvement, and AZT doesn't seem to be effective for much longer than a year and a half.

And how does the government respond to this crisis?

By sticking babies with intravenous sugar drips so they develop as many infections related to the IV as babies that are receiving treatment with intravenous immunoglobulin: Wouldn't want that nasty placebo effect to skew scientific results, would we?

By achieving homogenous sample populations for testing experimental drugs and then releasing them to women and children and people of color and present and former intravenous drug users who may metabolize these drugs differently.

By testing drugs against placebos for life-threatening disease where the best scientific result is having the control group *die* faster than the experimental group.

Are you convinced yet?

Okay, if I wait eight to ten years for good science to approve a drug, I'll be dead. That's simple enough, isn't it? It's tough being politically active from six feet under. If I remain silent in the face of this epidemic and the government's unwillingness to act effectively, then I'm just as well as dead. SILENCE = DEATH, get it?

But is any protest effective? Did political protest stop the Vietnam war, or was Nixon hiding out in his bunker, on his knees with Kissinger, praying for guidance? Am I a sacrificial lamb to a futile cause?

Here are a few other reasons for getting arrested at the FDA: I used to be a whore; now I'm a *whore for publicity*. I'm going to the FDA for the visceral thrill of being surrounded by the media. The camera bulbs flashing. The more people that get arrested, the more media coverage! And according to John Waters, everyone looks sexy behind bars. You'd be surprised. And who knows: I may be held for a week, and that way I'd avoid a wedding—that vile, hideous celebration of *heterosexuality* designed to *completely negate me*. Of course, if I had tix to the Prince concert in D.C. on October 11, I'd probably skip the demo, like one of Brad's friends is doing. *You see how complex the decision-making process is?*

True Stories, Part I

After Michael Morrissey was diagnosed as HIV-antibody-positive, his doctor told him that he should drink only one alcoholic beverage a week and avoid the sun. Michael was extremely fond of his preprandial cocktail. As a matter of fact, Michael was extremely fond of cocktails at any time of day.

What kind of vacations does that leave him? Should he go to the Land of the Midnight Sun in the off-season, when the bars are all closed?

Advertisements for Myself: The Whore for Publicity

Okay, I confess, the *real* reason I went to D.C. to get arrested was so I could write about it and *publicize* my soon-to-be-released novel *(Eighty-Sixed,* Viking/Penguin, January 1989, $18.95) to the *masses.* I planned on hiring helicopters and dropping *thousands of press releases* on the Names Quilt; I planned on leafleting the FDA, the police station, the FBI, the CIA, and any other governmental agency I could find. I would do just about anything to become *famous.* I planned to *seize the day* and write the homo version of Norman Mailer's *Armies of the Night* and be the *Great Fag Hope.* I was *willing to go to extraordinary lengths* to ensure my notoriety. But how could I possibly compete with the supreme male chauvinist of our time, in terms of vanity and vulgarity? Could I marry someone, stab her, then write a book about it? Could I have a murderer paroled into my personal care and then have *him* stab someone, then write a book about it? Could I write yet another masturbatory fantasy about Marilyn Monroe and call it art? Could I learn to pee standing up?

My T-Cells

I keep forgetting to call my doctor for my T-cell results, and I keep telling myself, "This is not a Freudian slip." Normal T-helper cells can be anywhere from 600 to 1,500; right now my count is some-where in the penumbrous region between abnormal and nonex-istent. Every three months I call my doctor to hear the dispiriting news that my T-cells have dropped a statistically insignificant amount. I extrapolate: By the year 2020 I'll have a negative count. I complain to my friend Joe and he tells me he has a friend in Philadelphia with four T-cells. "He's given them names: Bob and Ted and Carol and Alice."

His friend, of course, is dead now.

I finally make the call, three days late. My doctor tells me he has good news. "It won't be necessary for you to start taking AZT yet." Somehow I've managed to misplace thirty T-cells in the past quarter: another statistically insignificant drop. "Oh, and tests in-dicate that you've been exposed [which I register as *infected*] to Epstein-Barr virus." My doctor asks me if I've heard of acyclovir, an antiviral that suppresses the herpes virus. Dumb fuck, read my chart. You've been prescribing it to me for the last year, twice a day. "Well, try it three times a day."

Burroughs Wellcome, the kind people who brought us AZT at approximately $8,000 per annum, markets acyclovir under the trademark name Zovirax. Burroughs Wellcome is the de facto corporate sponsor of the October 11 demonstration at the FDA.

"Oh, and you should avoid stress," says my doctor.

That's real likely, living in New York City.

But why do I persist in going to all these endless ACT UP meetings and rallies and demonstrations? I wonder whether I have some sort of death wish.

ACT UP

ACT UP was formed in March 1987 in response to yet another angry tirade by the indefatigable Larry Kramer, one of the found-ers of the Gay Men's Health Crisis. According to the credo recited at the start of every Monday meeting by one of the two facilitators, "ACT UP, the AIDS Coalition to Unleash Power, is a diverse, nonpartisan group of individuals united in anger and committed to direct action to end the AIDS crisis."

Every Monday evening at 7:30, around two hundred cynical queers both male and female meet at the Gay and Lesbian Community Center. Everyone is named Michael. For clarity's sake, I've given some of them pseudonyms. Periodically refugees from twelve-step programs meeting elsewhere in the building pass through.

Our logo is "SILENCE = DEATH": To remain silent about the AIDS crisis is to be an accomplice to death. We've covered the city with stickers: a pink triangle (remnant from the Holocaust: Germans made Jews wear yellow stars of David, and fags pink triangles) on a black background, with the logo in white. At demos and rallies we chant "We'll never be silent again!"

ACT UP has no leaders. Meetings are run according to a modified version of Roberta's Rules of Order and are democratic to the point of near anarchy. The facilitator's role is to try to allow as full a discussion as possible without letting things slide into complete chaos, and to lower the level of vituperative and personal aggrievement to an acceptable level.

Yet somehow, miraculously, things get done.

ACT UP had its first protest on Wall Street in the spring of 1987, stopping traffic at seven in the morning and hanging Frank Young (commissioner of the FDA) in effigy. "No more business as usual," we chanted, protesting the exorbitant price of AZT (then $10,000 a year). Seventeen were arrested at this demo. Since then, ACT UP has held protests at *Cosmopolitan*'s headquarters (protesting an article stating that heterosexual women were not at risk), at Kowa manufacturers (when Kowa in Japan stopped selling dextran sulfate to Americans), at N.Y.C. Health Commissioner Stephen Joseph's office (protesting municipal AIDS policies), at both the Democratic and Republican conventions, and hounded the Presidential Commission on HIV relentlessly.

But why are there so many crazies at ACT UP? And why are the paranoid ones the loudest? Vocal members include one-note maniacs like the members of the International Socialist Organization who respond to every issue like presidential candidates at televised debates by ignoring the question at hand and with the most tenuous association segueing into a canned speech; the AZT-is-poison lobby; the paranoid-government-conspiracy contingent; the radical with lips thicker than Sandra Bernhard's who endlessly organizes kiss-ins; the self-proclaimed fattest and loudest megalomaniac who, in profile, bears a marked resemblance to Al Sharpton; the person of color who is constantly expressing extreme umbrage at any imagined slight; the fabulous dancer with the dazzling dangling earrings; the voice of Compassion, an out-of-work actress with a penchant for grandstanding with humor, who appeals to our deepest emotions and rarely our intellects (is this an *audition*?); the slender young cutie who demonstrates for the masses the latest fund-raising T-shirt on his own body; the Muscle Queen whose hopeless erudition continually mangles the English language (why can't he just flex silently?); the Religious Fanatic who exhorts us in passionate sermons to perform acts of civil disobedience at St. Patrick's Cathedral after Cardinal O'Connor tossed Dignity, a gay Catholic group, out of the church (why doesn't he just leave the Catholic faith, and what does this have to do with AIDS?); the radical with snot dribbling down his nose, screaming for more beds (there's one waiting for him at Bellevue); the Voice of Reason; the Voice of Sarcasm; the Voice of Roberta Herself (an activist who spits out Robert's Rules of Order by rote, letter-perfect); the Voice of Bitter Irony; the Voice of Despair; the Voice of Righteous Anger; the Voice of Utter Madness; and several other affective disorders as yet unclassifiable in the general scheme.

Sometimes I wonder, if I had a boyfriend, would I bother with the endless Monday meetings? I'm an ancient fossilized nightmare on the other side of the age of trust (i.e., thirty-plus): too old to rock and roll and too young to die. What am I doing in the midst of all of this youthful energy, these cute radicals? By the time the meetings are over at ten-thirty I'm too exhausted to cruise and I just want to crawl back into my coffin.

I go to the Monday meetings and about half of the demonstrations, and once I even went to a poster party on a day when it was around fifteen degrees above zero at some dyke's apartment in Tribeca (she didn't have a buzzer and she was on the phone for fifteen minutes so we froze in the winter wind until she hung up and let us in), where we made posters for a demo and I was chastised for being messy. *I should be doing more.* I am totally suffused with Catholic guilt, despite the fact that I was born Jewish.

At the Monday-night meetings, we plan actions and zaps, vote on expenditure of funds for our activities, and have endless arguments over procedural matters and AIDS-activist theory. We also have elections (the old high-school popularity contests) for facilitators (it's important to have decorative elements to look at during procedural matters). A cute but inarticulate fag wins by popular acclaim, followed by a mysteriously well-liked dyke. The sage and acerbic feminist who remarked in her statement that being a facilitator was "the closet thing to having my own talk show" collects several votes. We discuss whether to incorporate as a nonprofit organization for an hour and a half on a day when both temperature and humidity top ninety, before eventually tabling the matter until Halloween. The sexy socialist from the ISO with the tight, well-worn jeans ripped in just the right places says he isn't going to pay taxes to murderers, but then, what would you expect a commie pinko fag to say? We spend hours debating the merits of whether national health insurance should be one of our basic demands on every flyer we send out. We spend moments discussing whether we should start every meeting with a kiss-in.

We have a heated debate about whether to include a person of color and a PWA (Person With AIDS) whenever we send representatives to an AIDS-activist conference or a meeting with officials. I have trouble with the parity and quota system. I mean, when they talk about people of color, who am I, *Mister Cellophane*? Am I colorless, odorless, transparent, and lethal? So say some of my exes. And can I even ask these questions without being accused of sexism, racism, xenophobia, and homophobia?

I kibitz with pals on the sidelines, exchanging sarcastic comments during the Monday-night meetings. Cynicism generally sets in after eight months of involvement with the group.

My Larry Kramer Problem

Larry Kramer has this annoying habit of founding organizations and then renouncing them. It would be easier to treat him as the Lyndon LaRouche of the gay movement, another member of some insane fringe, and simply ignore his rantings and ravings as those of a demented lunatic. Unfortunately, beneath the spleen and venom, he usually is right.

Ten years ago he wrote an amusing novel called *Faggots* about homos doing the disco-gym–Fire Island circuit and fornicating like bunnies. The moral of the story being that this wasn't particularly healthy emotionally, and it would be better to have relationships of a deeper resonance. Of course, he was immediately attacked in the pinko fag left-wing press for being anti-sex, a moral puritan.

And now I suppose if we had all taken his advice and stopped having sex with more than six thousand partners, we wouldn't be in this mess today. But to draw any analogy between the two seems the most specious form of logical analysis. I place it under the category of brutal irony and leave it at that.

Larry Kramer helped found the Gay Men's Health Crisis, which was originally organized to help fund medical research for a cure for AIDS. After considerable internal squabbling, which he documented in the thinly veiled *pièce-à-clef The Normal Heart,* a political diatribe in the guise of a play (in which he attacked Mayor Koch for his response to the AIDS crisis, and GMHC for its nonactivist behavior), he was ejected from GMHC. Since then he has written a series of screeching editorials in the *New York Native* and *The Village Voice* about the pitiful city and federal response to the AIDS crisis.

Larry Kramer spoke to gay groups on numerous occasions. At one talk at the Community Center he said, "Look to your left, look to your right. Half of you will be dead from AIDS in ten years. Why aren't you fighting for your lives?" He inspired a group of people to form ACT UP. But, once again, the organization got away from him. And after the six-month saturation period, he, too, became bitter and cynical. ACT UP, originally organized to speed up drug testing and treatment, had evolved into a democratic organization to the point of near anarchy and grown into two-hundred-member Monday meetings and a myriad of committees and subcommittees (Issues, Treatment, Prison, Election, Majority Action, Women's, Fund-raising, Media, Outreach, and more). Larry had offered to front the money for a fund-raising letter, so we wouldn't have to divert money needed for actions and demonstrations. Three months later he retracted his offer, with a bitter letter accusing ACT UP of losing its focus. He also chided ACT UP for not being sufficiently mature enough to spend the organization's own money on its goals. Indian giver. At that point it was necessary to find another person to write the cover letter of the fund-raiser, because who could tell if Kramer wouldn't publicly denounce ACT UP in three months?

The fund-raising chair read Kramer's letter with controlled fury and told us that, as usual, Larry had a lot to say, and we should ignore the tone and concentrate on content.

What I hate most about Larry Kramer is—his prose style. There. I said it. I can't read him anymore. Who does he think he is, Noam Chomsky writing about transformational generative grammar? That's the mark of a fag. Here we are in a life-and-death situation, and what am I doing? Rearranging the furniture on the *Titanic;* making stylistic complaints. The amount of chaff in his writing is so thick I can barely make it through his prose to get to his points. Somewhere along the line he lost his sense of humor. I don't know why losing a hundred and twenty friends and acquaintances to AIDS would do that to someone, but let's face it, it did. And now Kramer is consumed by so much anger that he can offer only venom and accusations. Larry Kramer—the fag that cried wolf, Cassandra, the prophetess of doom—shrieks his diatribes into the wind, and no one listens.

CD Training

Anyone who wants to get arrested must attend a civil-disobedience training session. Great. Another fucking ten-hour meeting.

At last week's Monday meeting, John told us that the FDA's public relations had asked him exactly what ACT UP was going to do on October 11. He replied, "We're going to take over the FDA. We don't think that it's being run effectively, and frankly, we think we can do a better job."

In the seventies, an earring in the left ear meant you were queer on the East Coast; on the West Coast, it was the right ear. To avoid semiotic confusion, to dispel all doubts, our virile leader, Gregg, wears an earring in each.

During the endless CD training, we go over the reasons for our siege at the FDA: because we disagree with the principle of placebo testing for life-threatening illnesses; because the FDA isn't releasing drugs fast enough; because the current three-phase drug-approval process is ineffective; because trials exclude women, minorities, and former drug abusers, who may have different reactions to these drugs; because the FDA refuses to accept foreign data, and a drug like dextran sulfate, which has been in use for more than twenty years in Japan to lower blood pressure, must undergo toxicity tests; because the bureaucracy is inactive; because the FDA blocks underground buyers' groups; because we want informed choice for treatments; and so on.

We talk about nonviolent civil disobedience (avoid physical abuse; don't carry anything that could be construed as a weapon; no verbal abuse to the police; if you're being beaten, don't fight back; get support from other demonstrators) and discuss the nonviolence guidelines that ACT NOW (AIDS Coalition to Network, Organize, and Win, a national coalition of AIDS-activist groups throughout the country) had agreed upon. We role-play blocking FDA employees from entering, explaining our position to members of the media, getting arrested by the police. Gregg tells us that there are degrees of noncooperation with the police: Once we are arrested, we can continue nonviolent civil disobedience by refusing to walk to the paddy wagon; refusing to cooperate with processing by giving false identification information; refusing to pay fines and bail. Gregg describes the process of action, police warnings of arrest, booking, arraignment, and trial. I am intensely distracted by a dazzlingly attractive youthful playwright with green eyes to die for, until he confesses to me that he's attracted to Brits.

The general plan for October 11 is as follows: There will be a moving picket line in front of the FDA. Some people will get arrested by crossing police lines. This least-effort mode appeals to me. Perhaps I can work on my tan. Others will try to break into the building, including Green Eyes. I consider escalating my radical quotient, then recall my completely Semitic background. Not worth the effort.

All those who want to be arrested must join affinity groups of ten to fifteen people, plus one or two support people. As an affinity group, we will decide our plan of action: Will we break into the side entrance and trash typewriters, steal files, write memoranda restructuring the FDA, make long-distance phone calls, drop buckets of blood on FDA Commissioner Frank Young's desk? Will we hang banners outside, sell illegal drugs, create a diversion so another group can break into the building?

Only three of us are committed to getting arrested at the action; the rest came to the training for information and for possible future actions. So I only have to go to every ACT UP meeting until the demo so I can find an affinity group to join.

Previous Entanglements with the Law

I've been to demos before—the Anti-Nuke rally in 1980, when more than half a million swarmed up to Central Park; the July 4 Sodomy March in 1986, protesting the Supreme Court's *Hardwick* decision, which said rights to privacy do not cover consensual homosexual acts; and numerous others—but I've never been arrested before. In fact, the only time I was ever arrested was back in Hollywood, California, in 1978. I was taking an old college roommate to the airport and we were late. My cheap Chevy-as-in-cheese Vega sat there at the light, left signal blinking, gears grinding, engine preparing to melt down. The light changed; the car in the approaching lane paused, as if to let me by. Grateful for the opportunity, I hung a quick louie and was on my way.

For years I have been afflicted with some sort of psychomotor-neurological blind spot that impairs my judgment. I cannot blame it on excessive consumption of mind-altering drugs; I guess I'm *just retarded*. The car in the approaching lane, which had one of those rotating red lights on the roof, flagged me down. It was a police car. I explained our plight and my misunderstanding. The officer was not amused.

Back in the seventies I was under the mistaken impression that I could operate under a different set of rules. Aliens stole my Buick: They were bound to beam me up at any time. No sense in carrying earthly possessions like a wallet, a driver's license, or a watch. My friend hopped into a cab, cursing under his breath; the brute cuffed me behind my back, had my car towed; dragged me to the station, threw me into the holding tank. My neighbors climbed in through the window and rescued me with my license.

So I wasn't exactly thrilled with the idea of getting arrested. I mean, some fags like uniforms and leather and authority and play-acting and nightsticks, but *it's not my scene*. For me, there are two surefire ways to lose an erection while I am jerking off: the police banging on the door at six in the morning, demanding entry; and a member of my immediate nuclear family banging on the bathroom door at six in the morning, demanding entry.

The Decline and Fall of Western Civilization

If you're not careful, calcification of the brain can set in as early as the age of twenty-five. It's when you stop listening to FM radio for the latest hits and tune into oldies stations. You hear the latest songs (rap, new wave, salsa, Urdu tribal love chants) and you just don't care! The arteries in your cerebral cortex have started to harden; the synapses shoot and miss targets more and more frequently. You're going down the tubes.

Well, you're not alone. The entire country has been going down the tubes for the past ten years. The world is overrun with incompetents: I'm only doing my job.

Look at SAT scores, discourse analysis, deconstructionism, Contragate, the fact that the American people elected Reagan not once but twice! You've seen those TV shows where one high-school student identifies the Ayatollah Khomeini as a Russian gymnast; another guesses that Chernobyl is Cher's full name; and a girl, asked to identify the Holocaust, brightly replies that it was "that Jewish holiday last week, right?" *Situation normal, all fucked up.* Ronnie Reagan says at the Republican National Convention that facts are stupid things. Bush mumbles about the safety of the blood supply at the first presidential debate with Dukakis. Meanwhile, the youth of America sit glazed in front of empty-vee watching Monkees reruns.

I'm not saying that ACT UP hasn't been besmirched by this appalling trend. Witness the buzzwords *empowerment, inclusiveness,* and (my least-favorite word in the entire English language) *demystification.* Rarely will a Monday meeting go by without the mention of one of these dread utterances, and every time I hear one *my skin crawls.* These nattering nabobs of negativity have got to go. They have too many goddamned affixes and not enough substance. I just hate empty rhetoric.

While I'm at it, I might as well mention that I'm getting a little sick of all of these equations, with my fucking math degree from the Massachusetts Institute of Technocracy and a job in the exciting field of computer programming. I mean, SILENCE = DEATH is quite effective. I even like ACTION = LIFE. But after a while it gets pretty annoying with flyers with headings like "SILENCE = GOLDEN," "INCORPORATION = ENTANGLEMENT," *und so weiter.* What is this, Orwell's 1984? War is peace, ignorance is strength, et cetera?

More Stupidity

The horrifying thing is that we are the experts. My friend McCully from Manhattan Beach, California, told me this story about a scientist who was writing a position paper about nuclear winter, ensconced in some think tank in Santa Monica, or maybe it was Toledo, Ohio; anyway, at the end of one especially stressful session, he felt a need to get another opinion, to ask the adults, as it were, and at that point he realized that he was the only expert in the entire world in his particularly arcane field. *He was the adult. There were no other adults.* He couldn't have been older than forty.

Is that what empowerment means? Or is it merely the existential anxiety one feels when faced with the uncertainty of the future and the knowledge that one is responsible for one's actions?

It's scary to find out you are as smart as the media, as smart as the opinion-makers. One fine day, just for the hell of it, the Jewish media conspiracy decided to make Vanna White a celebrity, just to see if it could be done. And it worked.

So in the Soviet Union, the official disinformation is that AIDS is caused by experimental germ warfare by the United States government that somehow got out of hand. Luckily, in the U.S., we're too savvy to believe this explanation, aren't we?

And back in New York City, our Commissioner of Health decides that there are only 50,000 homosexuals infected with HIV, as opposed to the previous estimate of 250,000. This was done using a simple ratio of infected San Francisco fags over dead ones. Solve for x. But the infection rate was estimated at 50 percent, and I have personally slept with considerably more than 100,000 New York queers (okay, maybe a few were tourists) *in just the past six months.* Does this make any sense? Back in the fifties, Kinsey came up with a conservative estimate that 10 percent of the male population is gay; that gives at least 600,000 fags in New York City. And N.Y.C. is a major metropolitan area with a special appeal, drawing homosexuals like NoPest strips draw flies. So you would have to assume an infection rate of less than 8.33 percent. And with these new estimates, maybe the public at large is going to stop paying attention to the health crisis. Are we just being paranoid when we distrust these figures? You figure it out.

In October *Scientific American* has an AIDS issue, with a review of Randy Shilts's *And the Band Played On* by someone from the National Institutes of Health. It wasn't particularly favorable. But isn't that like Josef Mengele reviewing the Talmud, or Richard Nixon reviewing *All the President's Men,* or Prime Minister Pieter Willem Botha reviewing *Biko*? What would you expect? Praise?

Memories of Underdevelopment

Two weeks before the demo the incredibly glamorous Susan Sarandon (millions of lesbians and heterosexual males performed acts of self-abuse inspired by her breasts) visits ACT UP, offering moral support. She will be working at a fashion benefit for several AIDS groups, possibly including our own. Susan wears a low-profile, low-star-wattage outfit—an army-surplus jacket and jeans; yet she is a true goddess in our midst, our Kewpie-doll heroine. My local media experts tell me that she recently appeared on "Letterman" wearing a SILENCE = DEATH button: courage in the face of sarcasm and ridicule. The following day she goes on "Good Morning America" and talks about the planned action at the FDA.

Susan leaves to applause! acclaim!—and *not a moment too soon*. The evening's meeting quickly degenerates into the usual chaos. The two newest facilitators, elected last week to thunderous applause, allow the meeting to disintegrate into complete anarchy. Today has been one long demonstration: a protest at noon at the Waldorf against a Republican campaign fund-raiser with Reagan present; a rally a four at Sheridan Square called Gays of Rage, modeled after the black community's Days of Rage, against racism; and the regular Monday-night meeting at 7:30.

I went to the Waldorf demo. NOW was picketing around the corner; several gender-fucking fags pick up "I'M A WOMAN AGAINST BUSH" stickers. We carry signs: " _____ KILLED BY GOVERNMENT NEGLECT" or "_____ STILL ALIVE DESPITE GOVERNMENT NEGLECT." We fill in the blanks with Magic Markers. That's how I find out that Neil B. is dead. So that's why he didn't answer my phone calls. Boy, am I bummed out. The same thing happened in the spring when the New York Memorial Quilt was displayed in Central Park, and last year when the Names Project was in D.C. I'd see names of people I didn't even know were sick. In San Francisco, people come across names of friends they haven't seen or heard of in years in the obits of the *Bay Area Reporter*. I feel like punching out the nearest government official. I want to deck the entire Department of Health and Human Services. Why are they killing us through government inaction?

I don't know about the rest of you, but I can take only one

demonstration a day. I have this limited tolerance for activism. I also have this job that appears to be more tenuous every day. They know I haven't been paying attention for the past three years. Nonetheless, I must keep up the facade. This requires my physical presence in the office—in most cases, a necessary and sufficient condition to retaining gainful employ at this establishment. So after the requisite two-hour lunch, I return to work, and skip the Gays of Rage demo. People are testifying in Sheridan Square about their personal experiences of anti-gay violence. It's fall in the Big Apple: open season for fag-bashing. Several queers have been beaten, and a few have been killed in the past few weeks. But it's not really my style. If I wanted to hear personal testimony, I'd go to a twelve-step meeting, join a Baptist revival church, or buy *People.*

So by the time the meeting starts, a lot of people are all fired up and ready for action. The new facilitators, elected chiefly for decorative value, are no match for tonight's rabid brew.

A member tells us about the Names Quilt fuckup. Cleve Jones is bringing the Names Memorial Quilt to Washington on Columbus Day weekend, a few days before our planned demo. He had applied in January with the National Parks Service to display the Quilt on the Mall. Due to the summer drought, the Mall has been closed for resodding. The Ellipse is the only other outdoor location large enough to display the ten thousand panels of the Quilt. But the Parks Service has committed the Ellipse to the Ukrainian Millennial Society, which is celebrating a thousand years of Christianity in its homeland. The Ukrainians had applied for their permit only three weeks ago. ACT UP will flood the phone lines to the National Parks Service until justice is done!

The Issues Committee announces seventy-three more FDA teach-ins.

The Media Committee tells us that ACT UP/ACT NOW has received great media response thanks to our press kits. The FDA takeover is even mentioned on the front page of *USA Today.*

Our resident megalomaniac tries to disrupt the meeting for an impromptu demo, a continuation of the Gays of Rage. With inflammatory rhetoric reminiscent of a certain reverend associated with the Tawana Brawley case, the demagogue exhorts the group to leave and stop traffic on Sixth Avenue. "We have enough people here to really make a statement. We know that there are policemen attending this meeting. We have to leave right now!" A member dashes out, and Megamouth accuses him of being an informer. Energy is high. Blood is boiling. I am mad. I can focus on only one issue at a time. I'll deal with fag-bashing after AIDS is cured, thank you. What does this have to do with AIDS? The facilitators, buffeted about by angry rhetoric in this baptism by fire, barely regain control. The meeting will continue with important business until ten; at that point, members may leave for the demo. Megamouth whines (if it is possible to whine at 150 decibels) that we have to seize the moment, and by ten the police will be there. Was there a vote? Just some more virulent discussion.

The local coordinator of the FDA action leads the group in our "Seize control" chant. Rumors are flying left and right. "Is it true that the Health and Human Services demo is off?" *No.* "I heard that ACT UP/Boston is pulling out of the demo." *No.* "Is it true that there's no more housing available in D.C.?" *No.* ACT NOW is having a lot of problems reconciling the different AIDS-activist groups. ACT UP/N.Y. was behind the FDA action; the HHS demo was added at the request of L.A. and S.F., to broaden our goals for maximum inclusiveness. I imagine that ACT NOW's meetings are just as disruptive as ACT UP's.

Someone asks the facilitator to repeat the demand: "If there is any on-duty member of the police, the Federal Bureau of Investigation, or any other law-enforcement agency, you are required by law to identify yourself." *A policeman identifies himself.* We never expected this to happen. The meeting continues. There were no contingencies. We're all so tired and jaded, it doesn't matter anymore. The meeting ends at ten. Half of the group leaves en masse for Sixth Avenue, blowing whistles, shouting slogans, screaming chants. Is this any different from our other demos? Only that as a purely spontaneous demo, an unplanned event, it is unchanneled rage, unfocused anger—the closest thing to a lynch mob. Wanting no part of this, I turn left and head for the subway instead.

True Stories, Part II

Robert started crying at lunch because his cat was dying of gingivitis, and Robert's blood counts were off and his doctor had him take the HIV test and he was certain that his doctor would tell him that the good news was that he was antibody-negative but the bad news was that he had leukemia like his father, and of course Robert was exactly wrong in this particular circumstance, which is to say that he didn't have leukemia and he was antibody-positive, and what could I do but tell him that, listen, he could fall off the face of this earth and I wouldn't blink an eye, I'd just continue shoveling down my pasta primavera; a Mack truck could go out of control, mow down several hundred pedestrians, and crash into a plate-glass window, and I would just step over the bodies on my way to the men's room and deduct five percent from the tip, annoyed at the lack of decorum. You won't get any sympathy from me. I mean, back in 1981, when the first person died, it was something different. Maybe then it was like *Love Story* and tragic and dramatic and poignant and full of pathos and grief. But now that everybody's dropping like flies, who even notices? This is not an attention-getter. This is everyday life.

The Homo Conspiracy

I was sworn to secrecy; I'm not supposed to tell anyone about the Homo Conspiracy to take over the world, but life is cheap and so am I. So here's the deal: After we've recruited every Boy Scout and junior programmer analyst, we're going to place the breeders in camps, with constant disco music, which will either drive them crazy or bring them over to our side.

These are our plans: We're going to poison the blood supply. We're going to tattoo William F. Buckley, Jr., on his hindquarters with a branding iron. We're going to butt-fuck Dannemeyer and then toss him into a concentration camp. We're going to chug-a-lug Drano and hemorrhage on the Commissioner of Health's desk. We're going to slit our wrists and spurt blood from the jugular on the mayor. We're going to scarf down our favorite diuretics and piss on City Hall; we're going to mainline horse and vomit in front of the President; we're going to jerk off on the Pontiff's personalized toilet seat.

You've tried to get rid of us: Now it's our turn to eliminate you. Imagine a world without breeders. Homos and lezzies sit sipping cappuccino at a café on Bleecker Street. We have nothing to worry about: We have enough turkey basters to last us until the next millennium.

Or maybe we'll just disappear one day. Without us talented *fags* and *dykes,* Broadway will grind to a complete halt, there won't be a single restaurant left open in the tri-state area, and hair everywhere will be *completely unhinged.*

You can't stop us now: We already control all the major advertising agencies in the country; we've bought the media from the kikes. Sometime next year you'll turn on "Masterpiece Theatre" and watch homo love scenes. The kiddies will see condom commercials during the Saturday-morning cartoons. Lesbo newscasters will eat pussy during the six o'clock news.

Night of the Living Dead

Middle America is scared of us, an army of perverts, *and rightly so!* We are lethal weapons. We are not innocent victims. We kill and kill again. The general population sees us as the walking wounded, an army of lepers, infected with the virus; they will wear their elbow-length yellow-rubber gloves and carry night-sticks. And we'll shout back: "Gloves are for fisting, not arresting!"

The most frightening aspect to them, the enemy, is that we can pass. How can you tell if you are surrounded by fags? We don't lisp anymore. Our wrists aren't limp. There's no way to tell us apart from the general population because *we are the general population*. It's Night of the Living Dead, with pod people everywhere.

Imagine the bravest army ever. Some of us are sick; some of us are covered with lesions; some of us can barely walk; some of us are asymptomatic; some of us are healthy and lending our fullest support to this cause because we are fighting for our lives!

Apologia pro Vita Sua

Do you know why I am telling you all of this? Do you think I'm just trying to entertain you with these out-and-out lies? You couldn't be farther from the truth. I want to terrorize you. I want to spur you into action. I want to show you how fucking angry I am. It took five fucking years for President Ray-Gun to even say the word *AIDS* aloud. He tried to sweep the problem under the rug by creating a commission to come up with some recommendations on the AIDS crisis; he appointed some of the most homophobic and reactionary right-wing lunatics to this commission, including a Catholic cardinal; for a year, this commission met and held hearings, and with some helpful prodding by ACT UP, the commission actually came up with some reasonable recommendations; and what did Ronnie "Bitburg" Reagan do? Ignored his own commission.

I can understand how Larry Kramer self-destructed. It's too late for a rational dialogue with the government, when it responds only with delays, malice, and all of this talk about the "general population" not being at risk. I want you to be afraid of us. I have blood in my eyes and a fire in my belly and I am tired of watching my friends lose their minds and control of their bodily functions. At this rate, Europe will probably come up with the cure, but in the meantime there's a lot that the U.S. can be doing. The government lies to us every day. Tony Fauci of NIAID (National Institute of Allergy and Infectious Diseases) had to be up against the wall in a congressional hearing before he admitted to Congressman Ted Weiss, a saint in anyone's book, that he simply did not have the staff for the paperwork; aerosol pentamidine's approval for general use was delayed for over a year and a half because *he did not have the staff.* Why did it take him a congressional hearing to tell someone he was understaffed? Because there's no goddamned leadership and the President couldn't care less.

Flashbacks and Postmortems

It's the final Monday meeting before the action, and Bobby B. sings the new ACT UP rap song. Suddenly I find myself in the throes of a drug flashback (acid? isoprinosine? azidothymidine?): I am four years old, hands tied to the crib to prevent me from "touching" myself, totally *disempowered,* standing with the black-and-white TV on in the next room. It's time for "The Mickey Mouse Club" show. "Sing us a song, Bobby," chorus the Mouseketeers, and Bobby straps on his guitar, strums a few chords, and begins to sing. Bobby B. finishes his catchy rap and everyone applauds. I sit on my hands. I know, it's just professional jealousy. Why aren't writers ever so lionized? I don't want to have to become an alcoholic to be famous.

National Public Radio tapes our meeting.

The Quilt fuckup has been resolved. After four thousand phone calls to the Parks Service and negotiations with the Ukrainians, the Millennial Society had agreed to withdraw to the Washington Monument area and ceded the Ellipse to the Quilt, in exchange for the use of some of the Names Project's sound equipment.

Gregg of pirate earrings and swarthy sexuality tells us that the FDA has canceled most meetings for the day of the demo, and that employees are being encouraged to take the day off. "We have already seized control." He leads the "Seize control" chant again. On Wednesday, there will be the last pre-action meeting. My affinity group, a nameless ragtag collection of misfits and otherwise unaffiliated homorganisms (we had formed at last Monday's meeting; vanilla activists who wanted to be arrested for transgressing police lines), will be meeting an hour earlier.

One of the several thousand Michaels tongues me in the ear during the meeting and I lose my balance as a miniature tsunami crashes through my inner ear. Is this a proposal of marriage? I can no longer think straight.

Megamouth Michael gives a postmortem of last week's disastrous demo. One ACT UP member was arrested for assaulting a policeman, clearly a trumped-up charge: Faggots don't hit police, they just dress like them in riverside cocktail lounges. Megamouth was also arrested for disturbing the peace. Megamouth complains about rumors that some people are blaming him for inciting the group to do unsafe actions. To increase the level of paranoia, he tells us that the police are playing hardball now.

Stephen Joseph, the health commissioner, has been getting a lot of phone calls in the past few weeks; last Wednesday, the police woke up and questioned an individual at his home at five in the morning. Our legal-support team hands out a flyer titled "SILENCE = GOLDEN": We don't have to say anything to the police. It's the old "right to remain silent" clause. Some splinter group called Surrender, Dorothy may be behind the phone calls. "Don't call Stephen Joseph unless you're a close friend," we are advised.

I leave the endless meeting at ten for dessert: another sugar infusion and a caffeine injection.

Pornography, Music Videos, and Blood

I'm pissed about the timing of Wednesday's meeting: I'll miss the vice-presidential debate. I never watch television. I bought the boob tube only as an accessory for my VCR. I try to keep an even split between the adult and nonadult movies I rent. Luckily, PBS carries the debates an hour and a half later: It was doing live coverage of some Wagner operafest, and some of the divas had a mud-wrestling fight in the middle, forcing a delay in broadcasting the debates.

My affinity group meets in the pantry, with yet another Michael facilitating. In our disaffected group, this is pretty much equivalent to taking control. No one has any specific ideas. We just want a simple, vanilla arrest: to transgress police boundaries, get arrested, post bail or pay our fines, and be back in time for the evening news. Some of us are willing to get dragged off by the police, but only as long as the cameras are covering us. None of us is interested in dragging out the civil-disobedience thing to the point of noncooperation with the police, refusal to identify ourselves at the courts (or using pseudonyms like Tony Fauci or names of recently deceased PWAs): We all have gainful employ. We have a discussion about why we are protesting at the FDA and why we are prepared to get arrested. As with any group of more than three people, one or two people talk constantly for the sake of self-expression, and the rest nod agreement. Consensus is reached. Michael H. has devised a theme for our group: Tell Me Why. He has composed a list of around ten questions, like "Why has the FDA approved only 2 drugs when 130 drugs have proven effective against HIV in vitro?," and so on. He is going to make up signs with questions on one side and "TELL ME WHY" on the obverse side. Another member of our contingent volunteers to make armbands. And we have our own theme song, "Tell Me Why," by the Communards. Our support person, who won't be arrested but will track us through the legal system and carry our valuables and medication, hands us an information sheet to fill out. This is our second sheet: We filled another one out at the CD training session. I just love filling out forms. The form has the usual categories: home and work phone numbers, savings-account number, religious disaffiliation, hidden tattoos on buttocks and ankles, and so on.

The group meeting starts at 7:30. We get yet another form to fill out: The earlier forms have been discarded. I'm pleased that ACT UP/ACT NOW has effectively demonstrated the imitative fallacy by mimicking the FDA's bureaucracy.

Gregarious Michael asks us what we're going to do in less than a week. "Seize control!" is the resounding reply. We've already started to seize control. For the week of the protest, all FDA employees will be using photo IDs. Police will guard the entrances. There will be barricades on Tuesday. The woman in charge of public relations at the FDA calls Michael daily. The FDA is scared. It thinks we will be dumping bags of contaminated blood on the premises.

Peter shows a video of the FDA. We get handouts describing the physical layout from the Metro stop to the building. A sympathetic judge has volunteered to keep the courts open for us on Wednesday; Maryland celebrates Columbus Day on Wednesday, October 12. Nearby jails are overcrowded; the police may move us to a high-school gymnasium. Attracted by the fetish appeal of high-school locker rooms, several more members of ACT UP immediately volunteer to get arrested.

Another Michael rubs the back of my neck.

Stephen from the Issues Committee tells us about the Bush initiative, which we expect will be unveiled on Friday, to preempt our demo. This proposal theoretically should speed up drug trials: The FDA would give tentative approval to drugs after phase-2 trials, and final approval after phase 3. The FDA would be more involved in planning trials. On the surface, this sounds promising. But Stephen explains that it's just reshuffling the same deck of cards. Former debutante Anne, our media expert, demonstrates

the proper response for TV and radio. We shouldn't give thought-
ful and well-reasoned commentary: We should talk in direct, simple statements; we should talk in headlines. Anne supplies what is
destined to be the cry of the nineties: "It's a lie, it's a sham, it won't
work!" We all chant in unison.

True Stories, Part III

Peter was dead for a month before someone finally returned my
last message. We had both gone on our respective trips: He went
to L.A., and I went to Scotland. I suppose I received a postcard
from him postmortem. I called once and his best friend, Amy, answered the phone; she said he was very ill and that they were looking for a twenty-four-hour nurse; it was only a matter of time.

Dazed and Confused

My alarm goes off at 4:45 A.M. on Saturday. I stagger into the
bathroom and sneer at the mirror. Outside it's raining. I toss some
magazines I had gotten for the bus into my backpack. Search
for an umbrella. I've left my five serviceable umbrellas at
pornographic-movie theaters, art galleries, cocktail lounges, and
other disreputable venues: My sole remaining one is the pink fag
number. The bus shouldn't leave until 5:30; there's no point in being early. I decide to forgo the cab and take the subway for that
proletariat feel.

I'm not the only one subcomatose on the subway at 5:10 A.M.
The feds have cordoned off my car and declared it a fashion emergency. A woman in her forties, clad in a pant suit resembling a bad
Basquiat done on heroin, snores caustically. One man sleeps on his
back, reeking of urine. The rest have their heads buried at the
chest, against the window.

Cheery ubiquitous Brian from the Bronx is there, a bright
beam in the haze of radical somnambulists. No one should be al-

lowed to smile before 4:00 P.M. I put on my sunglasses and pretend he doesn't exist. Coffee is quaffed; donuts are devoured. People mill about aimlessly. I find a kindred spirit. The bus shows up an hour late. We file listlessly onto the bus, preparing to catch up on the missing hours of sleep. All is quiet, save for the lesbian in drag who converses with the certified hair-emergency about the eternal verities: relationships, therapy, and life after high school. I feel old, wizened, decrepit, fossilized. The driver decides to make us chill out by turning the AC on high. He yells at someone for opening the hatch. Why do we collect a tip for him at the end of the journey? The reflex of the two-dollar-per-person rent levied every Monday? Because we are incapable of cognitive action at this point.

Dentists are rumored to be in Washington this weekend, along with the Ukrainians. I wonder if some AIDS activists will organize a terrorist action to steal dental dams en masse.

Bamboozled into the Conference

The bus drops us off in front of a junior-high school. I'll be sleeping with radicals tonight. I've signed up for group housing in a seminary, instead of staying at a hotel, in order to undergo as many hardships as possible: living the gritty, sweaty, low-budget activist lifestyle. I want to take a shower and lie down for a nap. Unfortunately, group housing is unavailable until the evening. I have no other recourse than to attend the AIDS-activist teach-in.

I stagger to the registration desk, to find out there's a sliding-scale fee of ten to twenty dollars for the conference. No one from New York City was apprised of this. Raggedy Maria, surrounded by her ever-streaming hair, sits on the steps outside and says, "Don't pay it." Washington organizers grumble that if ACT UP/ New York had given them more financial support, the fee wouldn't have been necessary.

As we file into the auditorium (I've paid ten dollars, because I have no intention of going to the Sunday ACT NOW conference, which sounds as if it will be like an eight-hour meeting of ACT UP dominated by the radical fringe), two men hand us stickers that say "TOUCHED BY A PWA." Both side walls are decorated with large paintings announcing the "Why I Will Vote Essay Contest '88." Harried Heidi from New York, who was asked to speak a scant fifteen minutes earlier to preserve gender parity (because no women had been scheduled to deliver opening remarks), informs us of this fact irritatedly, and since she has nothing prepared, she bitches about the conference registration fee instead. This is the perfect opening for the two-day event. Contingents are battling in internecine warfare and the conference hasn't even begun!

A man from PISD (the latest acronym, standing for People with Immune System Disorders, created at the San Francisco ACT NOW conference a few months ago in the name of inclusiveness [the more the merrier!], a new subgroup of disaffiliated and debilitated, which includes PWAs, PWARCs (Persons With AIDS-Related Complex), People with Chronic Fatigue Syndrome, and People with Existential Ennui, among others) gives a rousing speech of unification and sexual liberation. He thrills us with his vibrant testosterone. I wonder why he doesn't give out his phone number. The stage is flanked by "SILENCE = DEATH" and "ACTION = LIFE" banners; the latter is ACT UP/L.A.'s flip version, pink on white, as opposed to New York's pink on black. Keep your sunny side up!

The afternoon is divided into four time slots; at each time, there are four sessions running. I go to a session on AIDS education. A California activist talks about the latest quarantine proposition on the November ballot. While we are stuck with demons and the figurative Lyndon LaRouches and William Dannemeyers, these poor souls have to devote all their time to fighting the literal ones. An educator from Eugene, Oregon, states that her hometown is the amphetamine capital of the world. Hmm, wonder

how much a roundtrip ticket to Eugene is. She is trying to edu-
cate gay men in her town about safe sex, but an estimated thirty
percent have unprotected anal intercourse in Eugene. Cancel my
reservation. After twenty minutes of general discussion, the
meeting is broken into three submeetings by the facilitators, who
have had only two hours of sleep the previous night, because several participants are complaining that it isn't possible to get to her
or his particular issue in such a large setting. At that point, I decide
to constitute my own group and disappear. I fear I would be too
conspicuous in my silence. A few months earlier, at the San
Francisco ACT NOW conference, groups decomposed into
smaller and smaller groups, eventually disintegrating into elementary particles: quarks generally of the strange flavor.

I return to the auditorium, where a woman of color is speaking. After fifteen minutes she interjects that she didn't know she
was going to speak and apologizes for not having a proper presentation planned. I listen to the litany of outrages: Although 14,000
AIDS cases have been reported in Africa to date, a more realistic
estimate is 140,000; on the average, women die six months after
diagnosis, while gay white men last two years; currently AIDS is
spreading primarily through intravenous-drug users via contaminated needles and their sexual partners, drug-abuse treatment programs have not expanded to help stem the epidemic, and there are
no comprehensive needle-exchange programs in the United
States. She accuses the government of conducting genocide with
AIDS, as smallpox was deliberately spread to the Indians in infected blankets: This killed half of the American Indian population. At the end of her session, the room opens up for questions,
and it's an ACT UP/N.Y. meeting in microcosm, with commies,
pinkos, members of the Workers' World Party, socialists, and other
socialites; the solution is reached through petitions, revolutions,
and cocktail parties.

Some members from the ACT UP/N.Y. Issues Committee
conduct a one-hour version of the FDA teach-in. A cute blond

named Mark with a necklace of worry beads is surprisingly articulate as he wends his way through several decades of government
regulations and historical precedents. During a break, United
Fruit Company, a political-comedy group, does a few skits: A
preacher and four singers perform homilies to sodomy; a vampire
is killed with a wastebasket filled with used condoms; a drag
queen, mistakenly arrested at a demonstration, comes up with a
complete change of clothing from her clutch purse.

I scramble downstairs to catch the tail end of a session with
John James, who publishes *AIDS Treatment News*. A few radical
faeries sit interspersed with the rest in the cafeteria. You know the
type: beards and skirts. I'm falling asleep, barely conscious at this
point. John James praises Larry Kramer and Project Inform for
bringing the drug problem to the attention of the news. Someone
asks about the syphilis-is-AIDS theory, and the typhoid quack on
Long Island. Penicillin doesn't seem to work, but the killed polio
virus looks promising; unfortunately, the supply has been cut off.
The hottest drugs now are CD4 and ddI. I don't know what the
acronyms stand for.

A British Canadian long-hair in colorful tights talks about having to smuggle drugs across the border: The only approved treatments there are AZT and aerosol pentamidine. The word
empowering is used at least three times this afternoon. An activist
says that community involvement is empowering. I reach for my
gun. There seem to be three levels of commitment: politically acceptable (and tax-deductible) service and health organizations,
otherwise known as death services, underscoring the adage "the
only good fag with AIDS is a dead one"; alternative treatments
(holistic, guerrilla buyers' groups, etc.); and political commitment
(preaching to the converted, we are designated level three). As
usual, the White Middle-Class Gay Men bemoan the fact that the
political groups have so few members other than WMCGM: Is it
lack of interest? Poor outreach? And, of course, a non-white, non-
middle-class gay man in our midst takes extreme umbrage at this

remark; I make my getaway on the pretense of running to the john.

The bathroom (a stall-less toilet, a single urinal, and a sink) is identified by a sheet taped to the door, with the inscription "MEN" (crossed out), "BOYS" (crossed out), "MEN" (crossed out), "SAFE-SEX CLINIC—BRAILLE VERSION." The alternative gender's powder room has a similar sign: "WOMEN," "WOMYN," "WOMIN." At this point, I find myself in an altered state brought on by sleep deprivation: My interpretation of these events is necessarily deranged.

We are going to the seminary at 7:30. Unfortunately, the candlelight vigil at the Quilt is scheduled for 7:00. I sit on the floor and wait, passively, watching an attractive man in a leather jacket place a sticker on the floor. The sticker says "A GAY MAN WAS HERE." He appends by way of explanation, "But the conference was boring so he left." According to Susan Sontag, the only intelligence worth having is skeptical, critical, and analytical. I dig.

We walk over to the church. Luggageless, curious Michael joins us. He had gone over to the ceremony at the Ellipse and met us on the way back to the now-locked junior-high school. Michael tells us that some ACT UP members started chanting "Silence equals death" during the candlelight march. Michael tells us in wide-eyed amazement that gradually the chant spread through the entire march. Jesus Christ! I think to myself. *It's just a metaphor, for godsake.* It wasn't meant to be taken literally. But some people just can't keep their goddamned mouths shut for five minutes without bursting into some chant.

We are staying in the basement of a church, which has dormitory bunk beds and several showers. There are enough beds and couches for everyone; unfortunately, we're short on sheets and pillowcases. Charlie from Toronto makes an emergency run for bedding. I join a group of hardy rebels for a quick dinner, thinking I will collapse at ten. But we wait for news from Charlie. We finally leave at ten, when I'm just about to pass out from exhaustion. After a seemingly endless Metro ride and an equally taxing walk, we arrive at an Ethiopian restaurant, where we wait another half hour for Charlie. I pause to savor the oxymoronic irony of Ethiopian restaurants. I've seen too many posters for famine relief. Another Michael defends Megamouth during our hearty repast. "He's not afraid of looking silly to make a point."

"But exactly what is his point?"

I'm too tired for cynicism.

We return by late-night cab. I stagger to bed, an upper bunk. Beneath me a woman sleeps. Eleven frazzled radicals are sleeping in this room. Someone asks me my name, shortly before I lose consciousness. "I like to know the names of the people I sleep with." How eighties. I sigh, remembering the old days.

Making Out on the Names Quilt

On Sunday I fall madly in lust with a Californian named Bill. Bill's former lover died of AIDS four years ago; his current lover's former lover died of AIDS three years ago; his current lover has ARC. Love among the ruins. If only I had an attention span sufficiently long enough to have a lover. As an act of social disobedience we make out on the Quilt.

The Names Quilt covers the equivalent of seven football fields on the Ellipse. Three-by-six panels—ranging from simple, touching, and heartbreaking to campy and outrageous—memorialize the dead. They range from a plain sheet of fabric with a Perry Ellis label to an elaborate sequined piano for "Watermelon Diet" Liberace. Even Roy Cohn, the most evil queen who ever lived, is remembered with several panels.

The first time I saw the Quilt, a year ago in Washington, I was blown away by it. Every panel represented a human life. Some panels were created by community and social groups for all their members who had died. Now I avoid looking for specific panels, except for my good friend Glenn Person, who died in '86. There are two panels for Glenn.

The most painful quilts are in the center. They are blank sheets of cloth, with Magic Markers for people to leave messages. By chance, I happened to see a message written to John Tannenbaum. "We're sorry you didn't know how much we loved you; we wish you hadn't decided to go so soon." John's lover died last winter. He had tried to commit suicide twice. Then John came down with AIDS. He succeeded on the third try. If at first you don't succeed . . .

I don't want to see the names of people I know anymore. I don't want to see any more panels with "I miss you unkel" written in crayon. I don't want to see my future in a patch of cloth, three by six feet. I don't want to see any more panels, period.

Hard as I try to make my self cold, harsh, cynical, invincible, I break down and cry anyway. Bill hugs me to comfort me, and we end up making out.

After a bizarre nap with my boyfriend-in-training, we have dinner at a truly horrifying restaurant in DuPont Circle that specializes in exotic margaritas. Then, drawn by the ineluctable attraction of the print media, we go to the local homo bookstore. I fantasize where my soon-to-be-published novel will reside. Oh, my God, there's someone from New York whom I'm supposed to be having an affair with. I duck to the lezzie section and am safely hidden by feminist tracts against pornography, instructional material on vaginal fisting, and home-repair manuals.

Bill tries to convince me to spend the night, but I have to be back with the radicals, and The Last Metro leaves at midnight. A peck on the cheek, an exchange of phone numbers, and I enter the endless escalator into hell.

A Virus of Unknown Origin ... DEATH: The ULTIMATE SIDE EFFECT ... A Feeding Frenzy of Lips ... More Dissension

Monday I show up at the rally at the Department of Health and Human Services. Rumors of dissension course through the amassed crowd like a virus of unknown origin. Word is that officials are already closing the FDA; perhaps, having accomplished our goal, we should try to take over another federal building. ACT UP/N.Y. may secede from the action. My blood begins to boil again. Does anybody think that any press people will be present anywhere else? Remember our goals.

At the rally, Reagan and his administration are tried in effigy. A prostitute from COYOTE presides as judge. Several people testify for the prosecution, including the eminently inspiring and impassioned Vito Russo, my personal hero. Vito has been a radical activist since Stonewall. Vito gives a slam-dunk speech. He had been diagnosed three years ago. He says his parents think that the government is doing everything it can, and that he will die. Well, says Vito, they're wrong about both. Vito excoriates the government for its inaction and homophobia; he blasts the far right and far left for trying to co-opt the AIDS-activist movement for its own ends. Someone tells me that was a pointed reference to the disastrous ACT NOW conference yesterday, which disintegrated into the usual brio of chaos and entropy. Vito concludes with a reminder that eventually the AIDS crisis will end; and that we must fight to change the system and ensure that the government will never fuck us over again.

After the rally concludes (the administration is judged Guilty! Guilty! Guilty!), the New York contingent meets at the flagpole. Mother Courage takes the spotlight, standing on a concrete embankment. We are here to center ourselves, she tells us. We are here to act in unity. We are here to discuss rumors that some New York affinity groups are splintering off. Representatives of each of the groups speak in support of demonstrating at the FDA, whether the facility is closed or not. One brown-haired rebel announces his intention to go to the FDA "because we made up all of these neat T-shirts" that wouldn't make sense anywhere else.

We end our nontraditional Monday meeting with a kiss-in that devolves into a virtual feeding frenzy of lips.

The Absolutely FINAL Very Last SWEAR-TO-GOD-ALMIGHTY-ON-A-STACK-OF-GUTENBERG-BIBLES Pre-Meeting

We convene at All Souls' Church at 7:00 P.M. for another endless meeting—this, the last pre-meeting before the demo. My friend David from Berkeley begs off; he has to take a nap. He'll be having dinner with a lubricious letch from D.C. and a bespectacled wuss from N.Y.C. Michael attempts to lure me to dinner; the letch entices me to his apartment. I can't. I'm here in a professional capacity. I need to suffer in the worst way. Frank the letch threatens me with piano bars, a well-taken point. What could be more dreadful? Not even a ten-hour meeting of rabid radicals. If I weren't Jimmy Olson Cub Reporter, I'd probably be in bed, buggering someone (or vice versa). So much for the sacrifices one makes for ART.

Paul Monette, famed author of *Borrowed Time* and *Love Alone*, flashes his press-release smile; he looks just as beautiful as in his jacket photo. Michael the Curmudgeon has seen him four times already: at the Quilt, at the candlelight vigil and march, on the street, and at the Smithsonian. Jersey Jon has run into Al Parker several times over the weekend, but what could he say to him? "I've admired many of your films. I especially liked the subtle nuances of your performance in *Fraternity Fuckholes*."

It's a typical meeting: logistics, logistics, and more logistics; applause at the appropriate intervals for those selfless individuals who have served the cause above and beyond the call of duty. The church is filled with angry activists. A group of extremely attractive men wear grizzled headbands like Red Cross bandages for bloodstained skull fractures, with red lettering on white stating "PWA" or "PWARC." It appears that the evolutionary intent of the human immunodeficiency virus is to uglify the human race: All the cute guys are dying.

The highlight of the evening is when the affinity groups introduce themselves and announce their plans for tomorrow. One group will be selling unapproved drugs; another will hang a banner from the flagpole. "Well, now the police know," remarks George the Wuss. "I guess they'll have to try something else." We assume the meeting has been infiltrated by members of the police and the FBI and various other subintelligence agencies. Three small affinity groups from Southern California, Arizona, and Nevada coalesce into "The Wild, Wild West." "Rats," I mutter. "Now they've got a theme song, too. We'll have to work on a secret handshake to keep one step ahead of them." After an hour and a half of the meeting, Saturday's keynote-address speaker from PISD stands up and announces that PISD is leaving for a nap.

At the podium stands an exceptionally cute facilitator named Mark, either Jewish or Greek or Italian, with short, curly brown hair and the bedroom eyes of Laura Mars. Jim Hubbard, famed cinematographer, auteur of the caustic documentary *Homosexual Desire in Minnesota* (the audience rioted at the initial screening, causing a sensation unsurpassed since the premiere of Stravinsky's *Rite of Spring;* several viewers slipped into irreversible comas, and most of the rest left in droves), tells me, "I slept with him in 1977." Thousands of times, I've heard similar declarations from Jim.

At around eleven, I leave with Curious George from N.Y.C. During the meeting, having skipped dinner, I'd scarfed down the sandwich meant for tomorrow's demonstration. But I'm still hungry. Activism is exhausting work. George and I stop off at a pizza parlor for sustenance and we run into three other rebels from California. It's truly a gathering of the famous and the soon-to-be, homo icons of the revolution. David from L.A. had written that groundbreaking celebrated treatise on jerk-off clubs that appeared in last week's *Advocate*. Michael D. had also slept with the cute facilitator, as had Michael L., another one of the knockouts from S.F. with the Red Cross headbands. Michael L. waxes nostalgic about the encounter with Mark. "It was exactly one year ago tonight," he says, brushing a crocodile tear away from his eyes. I wonder whether we should form an affinity group called Former Fuck Buddies of Mark. No. That would be unmanageably large.

Michael D., looped on his seventeenth beer, expresses dissatisfaction with the New York activists using subtle nonverbal communication. He grabs me by the neck and pins me against the wall. He tells me that the Californians are pissed with New York for sending out Harvey Fierstein fund-raising letters to their communities. He tells me that at the last ACT NOW conference they had confronted ACT UP/N.Y. with this, and that we had promised to adhere to their wishes. Then, two weeks later, they get another letter. They're also pissed at New York for various other reasons, which I won't go into here. I figure it's the Hollywood Wife syndrome. Larry Kramer founded ACT UP/N.Y., and we hate him; the other regional AIDS-activist organizations were inspired by ACT UP/N.Y., and now they all hate us; and so on. In Hollywood, as soon as you get successful, you drop your first wife and pick up a new one, because your ex remembers you when you were young and struggling and eating dog food, snot dribbling down your chin. Familiarity breeds contempt. Michael L. refuses to give me his phone number; I leave him with several copies of my latest press release.

Exeunt all.

Paranoid Dreams

I live in constant regret. I spend sleepless nights, atoning for the sins I have yet to commit. A path diverged in the woods; I took the road less traveled and ended up lost in the Amazon jungle for months. I read mysteries and identify with the murderer: There is always a point where after some irreversible action everything changes for the worse. I think, if only I hadn't poisoned my land-lord and used my Black & Decker power saw to chop him into pieces and then tossed them into my Cuisinart and pulsed fifteen times and then thrown the remains into the microwave and then disposed of the household appliances at the city dump, then I wouldn't be in this mess today.

It's just as bad when I watch "I Love Lucy." I must be the only faggot in the Continental U.S. who actively hates Lucy because I have this problem of overidentifying with the protagonists of half-hour network situation comedies; my former therapist said that I do not have a strong sense of self and am constantly merging with other personalities, and I'm always screaming at Lucy because she gets me into the most embarrassing situations, and I don't like be-ing embarrassed.

That night I have a dream, a horrifying premonition, a mystical Shirley MacLaine out-of-body déjà-presque-post-pre-vu experi-ence. It's after the demo, and I'm in the hospital with a fractured skull, surrounded by fellow protesters, distorted limbs in casts, screaming for morphine and other painkillers. The doctor comes to my bed, shakes his head no, indicates that I have an inoperable anxiety. "I'm afraid we're going to have to triage this one," he says, stepping on the eject pedal at the foot of my bed. I wake in dark-ness, sweating; the strap beneath the springs on my top bunk has just snapped; my mattress could fall at any minute. I freeze. I see the headlines: "AIDS Activist and Unknown Author Plunges Three Feet to His Death, Smothering Lesbian in the Process." I stay motionless for the next hour. Groggily, the activists awaken. It's D Day. Markie takes a shower. I have to be peeled off the bed, clutching the frame tightly, like a hysterical cat up a tree. A slice of raisin-cinnamon bread for breakfast (no diuretic coffee), several unsuccessful visits to the john; and the grizzled, unshaven, unshowered-and-Aqua-Velva'ed activists are off.

The State of Siege

We fiddle with the passcard machines until we have enough fare to make it to Twinbrooks, Maryland. The train is filled with crazed radicals. "SILENCE = DEATH" stickers abound. The cute, crazed Canadian from the conference sings rude songs on the Metro about safe sex. A few seats ahead of him, a straitlaced woman wearing gold chains, a skirt, and sensible shoes chuckles. She takes out her spiral notebook and begins to question us. Facing the media at 6:10 in the morning. She's from the *Washington Times*. I have visions of glory and fame. Isn't that just like *The New York Times*? I give her my name, hometown, antibody status, and a brief explanation of why we are here protesting against the FDA. Three others join in, supplying her with more quotes. Then suddenly (the origin of consciousness in the breakdown of the bicameral brain) my cognitive powers are restored and I remember that the *Washington Times* is the local Moonie paper. But it's too late to retract! I can only hope the Koreans won't bother me back home. I decide to get another three locks for my door.

The two-thousandth Michael arrives with our signs. Michael brings the "TELL ME WHY" armbands. Jan, who suggested arriving at the Metro station at six-thirty (a suggestion I was vehemently opposed to) so we could greet our fellow protesters at the station in solidarity, arrives five minutes before seven, having shared a forty-dollar cab fare. How incredibly glamorous. I am momentarily distracted and utterly smitten until I see the pipe-sucking playwright pass by. Our signs have questions on one side and "TELL ME WHY?" on the obverse side. I choose the sign that says "WHY HAS THE FDA RELEASED ONLY TWO OF THE 130 DRUGS THAT SHOW PROMISE AGAINST AIDS?" We line the walkway with our signs, alternating questions and "TELL ME WHY." Periodically, we flip all our signs. After fifteen minutes, we're bored; we decide to go to the building and join the state of siege.

The Metro police arrest an activist who is in the process of spray-painting "SILENCE = DEATH" on the walls of the entrance to the station. There's the usual screaming and kicking. Activists surround the police, shouting "No violence! No violence!" Our group breaks up to watch the fracas. Then we reconvene and decide to stay together in solidarity throughout the day.

There are hundreds of activists at the FDA. We form a moving picket line and circle counterclockwise, inside another, larger picket line that is moving clockwise. I hope some news agency has a helicopter, for an aerial photo. We look like the goddamned June Taylor dancers.

An actions coordinator tells our group that there's a group by one of the entrances that needs some support, so we go over and join them. We don't really have much of a plan: We just want to get arrested, perhaps as a diversionary tactic in support of another group. Twelve activists have effectively sealed off one of the side entrances. We shout the traditional chants, create a moving picket line. Someone hands out hard candies. Gay activists always appreciate something to suck on.

Protesting can be boring. The twelve activists are pretty much stuck in front of the door all day. What a drag. I curse my lack of foresight. I could have staged an impromptu reading! Nothing beats a captive audience.

The Psychosexual Response of Nonviolent Protest

"Quick! In front! They've arrested a busload of protesters and they're about to leave!"

Rumor has it that someone had let the air out of the tires of the first bus an hour ago. But now the first bus is ready to go. Our affinity group dashes back to the front of the building. The bus has already started moving. Still holding on to our placards, we hurl ourselves in front of the departing bus. Twenty police clear the immediate path. The cops brush us aside like so many summer insects on their arms. I get the brilliant idea of running a few yards in front of the bus, then hurling myself in front. This is much more effective. Once again I'm dragged away. I do it again. I'm dragged away. Then, one more time. I'm probably getting the same rush you get from skydiving without a parachute. This last time, at least three affinity groups have joined to block the bus. For every foot of progress the police have to drag off at least ten protesters. The police confer and decide to wait it out.

Another activist tells me that this time it's for real. Should I give our support person my glasses and face the rest of the interminable afternoon looking beautiful but dazed? I don't want my glasses to get busted, but I have 20/10,000,000 vision, and that's in my better eye. It's so bad that I can see someone's penis only when it's, say, close enough to be in my mouth. I really don't feel like having the visual equivalent of a bad acid trip, so I stick with my specs.

I look around for my affinity-group buddy, Markie. He's a few rows behind me. One of our signs has treadmarks on it. It's hard to do this sort of thing with placards in hand. I've enjoyed the pure physicality of being dragged. I ponder on the psychosexual relationship between the errant, absent father and Mister Policeman. As I cogitate about the sociological implications of our actions, the group chants to the police, some of whom are wearing surgical gloves, "They'll see you on the news; your gloves don't match your shoes." We go through the usual litany of chants: "Frank Young, Frank Young, you can't hide; we charge you with genocide." "Test drugs, not people." After fifteen minutes it gradually dawns on us that we're not going to get arrested. A new chant begins. "We're tired, we're bored, we want to go to jail." Eventually the people on the bus, mainly from PISD, want us to let them go to the police station, now that we've made our statement. So we confer and decide to disperse.

Hours later, at the police gymnasium, I hear five women called the Delta Queens have blocked a bus for almost an hour.

"Who Do You Have to Fuck in This Town to Get Arrested?"

Peter has climbed atop the awning and set up banners that say "FEDERAL DEATH ADMINISTRATION" and "SILENCE = DEATH." He's setting off smoke bombs. He can't get arrested.

My affinity group goes to the rear of the building. We decide that we will divert police attention by stopping traffic, while another group attempts to break in the back door. We sit down in the middle of the street. Another group joins us, blocking the other lane. The police merely set up roadblocks at the traffic light a block away and divert the traffic. Hard as we try, we can't get arrested.

It's an odd reversal of priorities. The police are our adversaries because we want to get arrested and they don't want to arrest us. It's come to this: There are almost fifteen hundred of us radicals, kamikaze anarchists, lemmings with our "ARREST ME" stickers firmly stuck on our asses, just begging to get thrown into the clink.

I ask my friend Jim Hubbard, who is filming the demo for posterity, "Who do you have to fuck in this town to get arrested?"

A group of protesters break into the adjacent ethics building and hold a press conference. No one is arrested. We have a lunch break on the grass. Some of us lie down to catch some rays. It's around noon, and it feels like five in the afternoon.

We have completely transformed the building. The "RITE AID" sign in the ground-floor mall now reads "FITE AIDS." A "SILENCE = DEATH" banner hangs above the front-door awning. We've hung Reagan in effigy from the flagpole; his pants fell off to thunderous applause. An affinity group has set up a billboard showing the estimated deaths from AIDS in the U.S. Every half hour they blow a siren and the count is incremented by one.

A group is selling dextran sulfate, one of the many nontoxic drugs that the FDA hasn't approved. The Faggots and Dykes Administration has set up an office outside: They are issuing memos to streamline procedures and set up new regulations. They wear white lab coats with blood-red handprints on the backs. Another group has gravestone placards: When they lie down to be arrested, the visual message is quite effective. Some signs say "DIED DUE TO LACK OF ACCESS TO HEALTH CARE" and "DIED FROM RED TAPE."

At the main entrance are maybe eighty policemen.

In the building, quite a few employees spend the day glued to the windows, watching our cheap amateur theatrics. Most had gotten inside before seven. The building was sealed at around nine.

We decide to get arrested by sitting near the entrance of the building. Someone lets the air out of a cop car's tires. George the Wuss reports another vile rumor: We are going to be held by the police for three days. We are ready for our charge, but another Michael, who has a bladder the size of a subatomic particle, has to take one last piss. On the side of the building is a broken, unguarded window. What would we do if we got inside anyway? Make long-distance phone calls? Sneak into the cafeteria and put salt in the sugar bowls?

We break into a jog along the front of the building toward the main entrance. A cop tells us to move back, brandishing his nightstick, then dashing back for reinforcements. We are at the edge of the police sawboards at the main entrance. We shout our chant, "Tell me why," over and over again. I feel foolish. I wish we had the lyrics to the song and a voice like Jimmy Sommerville. At that point we realize that we can shout until doomsday and we won't get arrested. The police are a thick mass inside the police line. A group of protesters are being arrested for lying down at the entrance plaza; the police have circled them. Sylvia, a feisty grandmother, joins them.

We have to do something. We continue chanting our ridiculous chants. We have to make a break for it. Mild-mannered Markie, with his well-kempt beard and even disposition, lunges forward, under the sawbucks, and I follow. Suddenly we are in their territory. The rest of our group follow. The police tell us to move. "Tell me why! Tell me why! Tell me why!" we chant. Seeing a momentary lapse of attention, Markie lunges again. A policeman, angered, tries to stomp on his foot. We scream, "No violence! No violence!" The police calm down the angered officer. Finally, resigned, an officer tells us that if we don't move, we will be charged with loitering and obstructing passage and arrested. We go back to our "Tell me why!" chant. The warning is repeated and ignored.

I am the fourth to be arrested. A policeman tells me to get down on my stomach. I kneel, thinking he doesn't really expect me to take him literally. "On your stomach," he repeats. Well, if you put it that way. I comply. He handcuffs me behind the back with plastic handcuffs and asks me if I will walk to the bus. I tell him no, so *two* policemen drag me there. A cop takes my photo before sending me into the bus. Out of sight from any media, I walk up the ramp.

The charge is loitering and obstructing passage. It's ludicrous. We're sitting on the side. There are around sixty policemen blocking the entrance, and we're obstructing passage?

Eventually the bus fills up and leaves and we ride to a police gymnasium a few miles away. The scenery is delightful. The cuffs are a little tight. One activist complains that the persistent swollen glands beneath his arms make it even more uncomfortable. A sympathetic policewoman loosens his cuffs. Another rebel manages to slip out of his cuffs. Come on, guys, we're on the honor system here.

The entire experience feels so *punitive*. The sympathetic policewoman whom we've identified as Sapphic-leaning says that it's supposed to be that way.

In the Belly of the Beast

I couldn't sit down for a week, after the way the police brutalized me with their nightsticks and other similar large appendages. There I lay, making my one legal phone call to my dear friend Pussy in New York City to check up on gossip. "Hey, guys, I don't care if you brutally gang-rape me. Just could you keep it quiet? I'm talking to my dear friend Pussy." Okay, I'm lying again. We get processed. It's quite straightforward: There's no strip-search, no erections to hide. One cop gives me a satisfying pat on the stomach for reasons unknown. Yes, I realize I'm in shape.

After an endless wait on the bus (first the protesters on the bus in front of us have to be processed, and then we are called, one at a time), I walk down the ramp, accompanied by two escorts (as if I were going to escape), and enter a glass hallway lined with desks.

It's not as bad as I thought it would be. Sitting on the bus, I muttered, "I hope there's a salad bar." I had heard horror stories about bologna sandwiches on white bread with mayonnaise! I hope they brought in some brie for us.

At the desks, we are asked some basic questions to identify ourselves. The cops take another Polaroid of us. Then a policeman cuts off our handcuffs with wire clippers and we are ushered into the gymnasium.

We quickly set up a Genetian system, even though we're only in stir for about an hour. We figure out who the bosses are and who the punks are. I practice dropping the soap in the showers. I hope they requisition rubbers in the state of Delaware.

Fat Michael stumbles in ten minutes later. He tells us that the police wanted him to remove his nipple rings because they could have been misconstrued as weapons, but when he challenged them to take them off themselves, they deferred. It was all too horrifying.

I answer only to number 124, my plastic-handcuff arrest

number (124 out of 175, like a limited-edition print). The terribly self-absorbed playwright does a Feiffer-like dance in the gym, ending in a balletic swoon. I adore him and his pipe: It's so cute and pretentious to be under thirty with such freakish habits. I meet another gorgeous radical, an actor-slash-fashion-leader-slash-all-around-glamour-queen. I press my lips against him, hoping maybe to neck and pet above the waist at our next demo. I decide we will become lovers as septuagenarians, if we last that long.

Jan shows up on the next busload of cons. The gym floor is freshly waxed and gleaming. My wrists are red. Radical faeries do their celebratory and healing dances. Include me out. Me, I'm the one with the poison blow-dart for Tinkerbelle at the Peter Pan matinee.

We can drink all the water we want from paper cups by a cooler. Outside there are some Portosan toilets, behind a temporary chain-link fence set up for our benefit. We lie down on the gym mats. We're tired. It's around three in the afternoon and it feels like midnight. All I want to do is go to sleep.

Eventually, we are called by number to the exit. There we are given a violation form, and our possessions in a plastic Baggie. Outside, support people have pizza for us. The police provide a bus back to the Metro station. We ride back to the church. I shower and pack in fifteen minutes; then we grab a cab to DuPont Circle, where we'll catch the bus back to New York.

Return to Civilization and Its Discontents

After scarfing down a meal at Afterwords, Markie and I, laden with luggage, dash to DuPont Circle. The first bus has already left. Half an hour later, at eight-thirty, a bus arrives, careens to the curb. The crowd scatters. Transportation Michael (as opposed to Housing Michael) tells us to watch out for him: He's dangerous. There's absolutely no smoking on the vehicle with the bus driver

from hell. Markie and I climb aboard. I pass around my Halloween snack packs of M&Ms and Snickers mini-bars. Below us,
Mary Jane wafts through the aisles.

Again, we're in snooze mode for the trip home. Thank God,
most of the bus is comatose. No one is singing show tunes or
(worse yet) TV theme songs. Yet, three rows behind Markie and
me, a horrifying gabfest of enlightened teenagers ensues, the general subject being the meaning of life. A guileless boy admits his
desire to become a lesbian. Michael mentions that these are the
same ones who tortured us on the way down.

Freshly empowered from the day's valiant action, I stride man-
fully back and ask them, "Can you keep it down because some of
us are thirty and we have already had these conversations?"

The woman in the group retorts, "But I'm thirty."

I apologize. "I was only trying to be rude."

Startled, they gradually lower the decibel range. I return to my
seat triumphant, and fall into a deep sleep. I dream of the post-
action post-bus-ride meeting, to be held at the locked Community Center at three in the morning. Another endless meeting . . .

••

I wrote this in a frenzy of eight weeks, while I was waiting for Eighty-
Sixed *to be published. At Viking, it took about a year between acceptance
of the manuscript and publication. I was going crazy from waiting. I decided to plunge head-deep into a project dear to my heart. As I was writing
it, I sent queries to several magazines.* Rolling Stone *had already done
a piece about AIDS that year. The* Village Voice *had already published
a news account of the demonstration. Heedlessly, I wrote on furiously.
When I finally finished it, I showed a copy to my friend David Groff of
Crown. A year later, long after I had given up on this piece ever seeing the
light of day, he helped me get it into the inaugural issue of* Tribe, *a gay
literary quarterly published by Bernard Rabb of Baltimore.* Tribe *is now
defunct.*

*I was trying to convey a sense of ACT UP in 1988 by using the hy-
perbolic style of Hunter S. Thompson crossed with a queer Norman*

Mailer. To capture this energy, I tried to be as outrageous and politically incorrect as possible. Even as I was in the process of writing Queer and Loathing, I found myself disagreeing at times with the narrator. In the intervening years, ACT UP/N.Y. has evolved considerably. Consider this piece a fond snapshot of ACT UP/N.Y. during the heady early days.

Part
Two

Life
in
Hell

Etiquette for the
HIV-Antibody-Positive

As a well-known expert in manners, I was asked by the editors of this esteemed publication to compose a brief treatise on etiquette for the HIV-antibody-positive. I assumed this would be a relatively easy commission: I would consult various manuals and research materials and then I would rewrite selected rules and precepts in my inimitable style. To my dismay, neither the eminent Miss Manners nor the deceased Emily Post has written a definitive guide; moreover, Ann Landers and Abigail Van Buren have yet to provide even the most elemental suggestions. What follows, therefore, is a set of highly subjective rules, for which I bear full responsibility. In these uncharted territories of etiquette, I relied upon two signposts to guide me: consideration for your fellow (wo)man and common sense.

1. Avoid bleeding in public. Carry tissues with you at all time. Eschew handkerchiefs. In emergencies, a Kotex can come in handy. Hemophiliacs should consider carrying clotting agents.

2. Be sure to inform each and every sexual partner of your an-

Originally appeared in Body Positive, *Vol. 1, No. 9, September 1988.*

tibody status. If shy and not given to easy verbalizing, consider the compassionate suggestion of William F. Buckley, Jr.: a tasteful tattoo on the hindquarters.

3. Be prepared for the abrupt cessation of all activity when you announce your antibody status during an orgy.

4. There is nothing wrong with dashing across Sixth Avenue midblock during rush hour when the person adjacent to you sneezes; there is nothing wrong with refusing to shake hands with a bleary-eyed hay-fever victim. Henceforth, consider yourself an extreme hypochondriac. If you desire, cultivate this eccentricity to a high degree of refinement. Surgical masks are fashionable these days: No one should be without one in public. Similarly, elbow-length rubber gloves are rapidly gaining acceptance at cocktail parties and charity events.

5. Be considerate. When visiting squeamish relatives, carry your own silverware, bedding materials, towels, and works. If at all possible, rent a Portosan toilet for the weekend. Try to avoid informing your immediate family of your HIV status during stressful events: funerals, marriages, communal meals, or conversations. When the time comes, the use of sign language may be helpful in communicating this rather delicate fact.

6. Avoid sharing intravenous needles, toothbrushes, condoms, sticks of gum, crotchless panties, joints, ice-cream cones, dildoes, blood transfusions, wombs, tampons, zucchinis, and other intimate apparel.

7. It is considered gauche to inform a sexual partner of the not-so-recent past of your antibody status over the phone. Invite him or her to brunch. Slur your secret over the seventh cocktail.

8. Refrain from excessive cruising at AIDS benefits. This is unseemly behavior. Stenciling your first name and your phone number on your tuxedo jacket shows an appalling lack of taste. Be aware that contrary to your past experience, the large gathering at the john during intermission does not necessarily constitute a "very active tearoom."

9. Bodybuilders and other narcissists should abstain from sweating at public gymnasiums. Louise Hay's self-improvement techniques may prove helpful at this juncture; otherwise, try Mitchum Five-Day deodorant pads. Carry your own towel; drink from your own bottle of Evian; should you have an urge to spit into the drinking fountain, swallow the phlegm instead. Avoid public showers, steam rooms, sauna baths, whirlpools, and other possibly arousing venues. At all times men and women should wear jockstraps, underwear, shorts, and sweat pants, in order to prevent possible escape of seminal and/or vaginal secretions.

10. Gloves are essential for supermarket visits. Produce may be inspected with a magnifying glass and calipers; avoid any direct physical contact. You may find yourself purchasing more disposable paper goods, perhaps against your better instincts of ecology and conservation. Money and/or food stamps should be kept in a sealed Ziploc storage-bag to minimize handling.

11. Floss frequently before your biannual dental checkup to minimize bleeding. Refrain from the reflexive reaction to bite your hygienist as (s)he inserts large objects into your mouth and instructs you to clamp down. A mild sedative before the visit may be helpful. Avoid gagging. Male homosexuals may find this instruction especially easy to follow. When instructed to spit into the bowl, take care to aim with precision.

12. Children in elementary school should refrain from scratching and biting during routine squabbles. A water pistol should prove adequate for most confrontations; in the event that this does not suffice, brass knuckles are usually sufficient. For extremely fractious situations, summon an aide, an instructor, a counselor, or a police officer.

13. When visiting the seashore, be sure to use an industrial-strength insect repellent to avoid transmission of the virus through mosquitoes. In certain localities and communities, concerned townsfolk may desire to drain local swimming pools after you immerse yourself in them. Do not draw undue attention to your an-

tibody status, should you find this behavior embarrassing and overattentive. Both men and women should wear inconspicuous one-piece swimsuits with maximal coverage, or, failing that, wet suits or Aqua-Lungs.

14. Shooting galleries should be visited during off-peak hours to minimize contact. Although passing the spike was in former years a symbolic gesture of conviviality and communion, henceforth you must completely refrain from this practice. Clorox bleach or sets of sterilized disposable hypodermics may be offered to the dealer as a gratuity. As always, spitting at the methadone clinic is unseemly behavior.

15. Prostitutes should use discretion in informing johns of their antibody status. It is inconsiderate to wait until a masochistic client is bound and gagged before telling. All sexual acts should be performed with the use of latex prophylactics and/or dental dams, regardless of the client's desires. Payment in full should be accepted prior to services rendered. If these simple rules cannot be adhered to wholeheartedly, the prostitute should consider a reputable trade school.

16. Hair should be neatly groomed before visiting a tonsorial establishment. You may choose to supply your own combs, scissors, and razors. An extremely considerate patron would also carry a water spritzer to obviate the necessity of a shampoo, a portable hair dryer, and a Dustbuster for fallen hair. Whenever possible, exotic styling and dyeing should be performed in the privacy of your home. This also goes for tattoos and the piercing of ears and other organs.

17. In general, be unobtrusive in public. For example, try to keep on hand at least one complete outfit when doing laundry: Don't wait until you've run out of underwear, and you are down to one pair of jeans with holes in provocative places. Don't fight over dryers: This may draw blood. Again, a sedative may be helpful before visiting the Laundromat.

18. Realize that, unfortunately, your health-care practitioner is

probably quite busy these days. Try to refrain from scheduling tests for T-cell counts more than twice a week. Avoid calling him or her with minor, trivial complaints. Hangnails are rarely fatal; that malaise you find yourself experiencing with greater frequency may be simple existential anxiety. Consider: Perhaps you are merely worried about the Bomb and nuclear annihilation and the abyss and the lack of meaning in a godless world and the fact that the only station you receive clearly out of fifty-seven stations is the shopping channel.

Remember, next to your penis or vagina, a positive attitude is your best friend. Good manners and a positive attitude go hand in hand. Conduct yourself with grace and politeness. A few years down the line, when a cure is discovered, you can return to your debased state of ill-mannered crudity. Until that time, however, it is important to remain a paragon of decorum.

••

I wrote this for the Body Positive newsletter. I've always enjoyed making lists. Several years later, my friend Jim Lewis asked me to come up with a holiday gift guide for the HIV-antibody-positive. My list was suitably tasteless: It included a case of Sustecal; a vase from Pottery Barn that could later serve double duty as an urn; and a lifetime supply of anything. Jim liked it. Everyone else associated with the magazine hated it; they felt it was too grim and inappropriate, especially for someone who had just found out his or her status. Jim had just started editing the magazine. It was important for him to choose his battles wisely. He killed the piece.

Notes from the Front Lines: Writing about AIDS

Kenny told me it was difficult to find an HIV–positive person to be on this panel. I spoke to one writer who didn't want to be on an AIDS panel because AIDS doesn't define him as a writer; his writing does. Another writer told me he wasn't given a choice; he was just dumped on an AIDS panel. So here I am, in the absurd position of being on a panel organized by someone who had written a less-than-flattering review of my first novel and has somehow neglected to mention this to me and has no idea what an unbelievably petty person I can be. I feel somewhat less legitimate than my other panelists because I'm as yet asymptomatic. I suppose the inability to maintain a relationship for more than fifteen minutes after orgasm may count as a disability. My disabilities are primarily psychological, and I had them long before HIV. My symptoms so far have been mild side effects from prophylactic drugs and diagnostic tests, and a generalized dread. Sometimes I imagine that I had a false-positive test in '87 and it's just a lab error or freak coincidence that my T-cells have been steadily declining

Delivered as a talk at OutWrite, the National Lesbian and Gay Writers Conference, on March 2, 1991; published in NYQ, *January 6, 1992.*

and that the slight fatigue I feel at times is hypoglycemia or sugar letdown or side effects from poison pills or depression or age or laziness or psychological stress, and as a result the value of x is decreasing, where x is the number of stops on the subway before mine that I am willing to get off to pursue a cute boy, and that maybe I'm taking AZT and Zovirax and pentamidine and naltrexone and Z-BEC vitamins and lysine and vitamin A for nothing and maybe I won't get sick and develop opportunistic infections and wither away watching cable TV once I finally get around to ordering it (I got a TV when I tested positive) and working on my posthumous Bruce Chatwinesque essays, and maybe I'm not HIV-positive after all, and I wonder if this is denial or one of those Twelve Steps to Hell that someone placed a banana peel for me to slip on, and then the voice of Bette Davis or Lynn Redgrave, if you prefer, booms, "Butcha are, Blanche, butcha are."

For the past five years I've been writing almost exclusively about AIDS: I suppose I've pigeonholed myself into another subgenre: There's the Latin-American school of magic realism, the post-Sadean body-mutilation work of Dennis Cooper, and my specialty, gay Jewish humor for HIV-positive men whose T-cell counts hover around 200. This is equivalent to the evolution from network broadcasting to cable narrowcasting. I'm sure this is progress. I think I'm indexed on some editor at *The New York Times*'s Rolodex under gay AIDS-related humor, having reviewed two books in that category to date.

I don't consider myself disabled, just disappointed. My doctor recommended I contact someone in San Francisco to get on a Chinese herb protocol. As usual I procrastinated. Then I saw Woody Allen's *Alice* and the effects of herbs on Mia Farrow. When I realized I might be able to conjure up Alec Baldwin as a former lover, I was all gung-ho on the idea. At my next visit, I told my doctor I hadn't gotten around to it yet and he asked me what my most recent T-cell count was; then he told me it was okay, my count was too low for the protocol anyway.

I'm another example of that odious bugaboo, a white male socialized in this patriarchal society, a mess of all the -isms that I combat as best I can: a sexist feminist, a homophobic queer, a racist honky, a self-loathing narcissist, an anti-Semitic Jewish atheist, a leaden prose stylist, with trace elements of looksism, ageism, and ableism. I believe a distinction can be made between sexual predilections and tastes and -ismic behavior: For example, a gay man who sleeps with men exclusively isn't exhibiting sexism against women in this.

I was at the gym a few months ago and a therapist who is definitely in the top ten on the *Billboard* chart of sauna pigs said, "HI, DAVE, HOW ARE YOU? HOW ARE YOUR T-CELLS?" and I said, "Fine," and he said, "I'VE BEEN DOING INTRAMUSCULAR ALPHA-INTERFERON FOR THE PAST TWO MONTHS, AND I FEEL GREAT; MY T-CELLS WENT UP THREE HUNDRED POINTS," and I said, "Great," and he said, "YOU REALLY OUGHT TO TRY IT; THE ONLY DRAWBACK WAS THE FLULIKE SYMPTOMS I EXPERIENCED," and I said, "I'll think about it," and then I fled to the gym floor and wondered whether he ever needed to use a speakerphone and thought maybe I could try to recruit him to ACT UP demos to lead chants where we didn't have permits for megaphones and wondered whether this was a new ism, internalized HIV-o-phobism, or just personal privacy or simply the desire to tell others one-on-one my seropositive status myself before, during, or after seduction attempts.

I once saw a panel where a black lesbian feminist spent her entire speech denying she was speaking for all black lesbian feminists. I'm embarrassed that on some level my work is just one prolonged apology, including this speech. I've felt fraudulent my entire life: At this conference, surrounding myself with writers somehow legitimizes the doubt that I am a writer. I feel spectacularly unqualified to talk from the viewpoint of AIDS symptomatic individuals. Nevertheless, I think it's important to self-identify publicly as being on the HIV-AIDS spectrum. It's difficult. I wrote a piece about taking AZT for *The Village Voice* biweekly AIDS column last March and told my mom about it so she wouldn't read it on page-six gossip columns first, and then the piece was bumped for a newsworthy item. It has been continuously bumped for newsworthy items and I have this dreadful fear that they will run this piece the week after I die. I wrote an extremely personal piece for *Fame* on AIDS drugs and problems with the system of drug development and approval; *Fame* went under with my article at the presses. I sent it to *Wigwag* and the next day I read *Wigwag* went under. If anyone knows of any bothersome magazines better left unpublished, let me know and perhaps I can sink them, too.

I'm wearing a Diseased Pariah button ("KISS ME, I'M A DISEASED PARIAH") given to me by *Diseased Pariah News*'s cranky editor to co-opt and reclaim a derogatory term, albeit with a black-humor smirk, much as "queer" has been recently reclaimed. I think it's great when bisexual women identify as lesbians, when straight men and women support ACT UP. I was initially somewhat conflicted when I found out an HIV-negative person claimed he had AIDS to a news reporter at an ACT UP demo last year: Was he cheapening the suffering and nobility of someone who did have AIDS? But in ACT UP/New York, we have made a conscious decision to say we are all HIV-positive if arrested so the police don't split us up. The HIV-negative person was acting in solidarity.

I'm living in prospective dread. Sometimes I feel I'm an accident waiting to happen. Maybe I'd be a more appropriate panel member in five years; maybe that would be too late. I could have a narrow window of vulnerability. Now I'm on the sidelines, vicariously experiencing symptoms through hospital visits, treatment and data newsletters, medical reports, and the *Physicians' Desk Reference*. I'm waiting in line for the amusement-park ride. I have that increasingly popular fantasy to booby-trap myself with dynamite near death and explode in anger literally and figuratively at Jesse Helms. I have a goal of getting five books out, enough to make a mark, although this is shockingly egocentric; I feel like a dog marking trees and fire hydrants for posterity. It is extremely doubtful that issue will ever result from my spilt seed, unless someone can ultracentrifuge HIV out of my semen. On the other hand, I know, like every other teenager (my psychological age), that I will live forever.

Certain autobiographical elements inevitably filter into my fiction. I try to deal with sex as honestly or dishonestly as I do in life. In *Eighty-Sixed* I felt it was important to be graphic about sex, since I was extremely graphic about that truly obscene subject, death. The Puritan in me consciously avoided the erotic: I didn't want to pander or arouse. I wrote the most graphic scenes with clinical detachment. Blame it on six thousand years of Jewish guilt. If I can't have fun, why should anybody else? My next book, *Spontaneous Combustion*, a collection of stories disingenuously marketed as neither novel nor short stories, follows the continuing saga of Benjamin Joseph Rosenthal. It contains several stories with strong sexual content. In one story, Benjamin has a relationship with a seronegative person. I deal with elements of disclosure, sexual risks, and safe sex here. Gays call straights breeders. I myself am a person without color. I'm sure we'll come up with a derogatory term for neggies soon enough: Aseptic? Hermetically sealed? Sheltered? Or maybe just shy. David Wojnarowicz and Phil Zwickler collaborated on a short movie called *Fear of Disclosure*, in which Zwickler on voice-over talks of a sexual apartheid arising between positives and negatives. Yet I certainly don't feel people have an unalienable right to have sex with whomever they want. It takes two to tango (or, in certain cases, more: Adultery requires at least three). The slippery paradox is that when you disclose your HIV status to someone mature, it usually won't make a difference; however, if you are responsible enough to disclose your status to someone whose emotions are stronger than his intellect, he will respond with visceral fear, no matter how safe the sex might be. I personally am annoyed at those who don't get tested now. People who say HIV doesn't cause AIDS might as well say that sperm plus ovum don't cause pregnancy. Those intangibles who aren't tested who don't want to have sex with those who have been are intellectually fraudulent. Yet every informed individual has a perfect right to make any decision she or he wants to.

I personally feel much more comfortable having intimate relations with someone who is HIV-positive. A friend told me that he would tell a prospective sexual partner that he was HIV-positive, but not that he had AIDS. There are levels of stratification: people who have sex only with blonds with T-cell ranges of 250–350 and penises between five and nine inches. AZT-phobes may have difficulty dating AZT-philes, much as carnivores do dating vegetarians. Characters in my stories use subtle ways of disclosing their status, by saying "I started going to ACT UP after I tested positive" or "My nebulizer's broken—may I borrow yours?" or "After I tell you I'm HIV-positive and you run screaming from the room, can I give you a sensual massage using only my tongue?" It's become just one more potentially disastrous secret to divulge to a prospective boyfriend, along with "I'm incapable of long-term relationships," "I have a lover," or "I live in New Jersey."

I wrote *Eighty-Sixed* under a generalized dread. I took the HIV-antibody test the morning that I delivered my manuscript to my editor, expecting a chance of one in a hundred of acceptance and slightly higher odds on turning out positive. After I got my results, I became consumed with the insane fear that the normal publication delays for such trivial things as editing, catalog copy, getting blurb quotes, selling it at a sales conference, and then getting advance orders from bookstores were all part of a conspiracy to delay so I might have a posthumous publication—books of the recently deceased sell so much more, and there's a lesser likelihood of an audit by the estate; no one would be constantly nagging to be taken on a publicity tour, and so on. Although earlier drafts of a few stories in *Spontaneous Combustion* were written before, the bulk of them were written under the malevolent cloud of HIV-positivity. The content appears to me to be the same anxiety-ridden prose.

Writing is hard enough without disability. I go through endless avoidance activities: dusting the plastic blow-up pink flamingos, checking for the mail hourly, cleaning ashtrays although I don't smoke. I even have a full-time job, programming computers and mismanaging personnel, exclusively designed to avoid writing. I was hysterical after dapsone turned my entire body into a five-foot radish. It is difficult to write a review of a Canadian novel for an esteemed publication that is due the following morning (not, as previously assumed, the day after) at midnight when discovering a crab louse that had somehow miraculously escaped three cleansings with A200. It is difficult to write notes for a session on disability and sexuality in a faraway city between bathroom sprints after drinking a gallon of Colyte flavored with sugar-free powdered lemonade, in preparation for a colonoscopy the following afternoon, another senseless diagnostic test undergone in the interest of better bilking the insurance mill.

HIV/AIDS pretty much covers the spectrum of disability: People can go blind, become paralyzed, get dementia. Some drugs have side effects of lowering desire. Robert Ferro wrote a beautiful scene in *Second Son* in which two men with AIDS simply slept together. In *Afterlife*, Paul Monette honestly described sexual dysfunction in a relationship between two HIV-positive AIDS widowers. Gary Indiana wrote of sex, desire, and neurotic fear of AIDS in *Horse Crazy*. In my book *Eighty-Sixed*, I wrote a reductio-ad-absurdum list of safe-sex guidelines in the age of anxiety. Allan Barnett's "Philostorgy, Now Obscure," which has the distinction of being the first story in *The New Yorker* with a gay man who has had more than two sexual partners in the past ten years, had a touching love scene between two ex-lovers, which for purely esthetic reasons didn't make it into the magazine. Peter McGehee's exuberant freewheeling sex in *Boys like Us* seems just like the old days, only now with condoms.

HIV/AIDS differs from many disabilities in that it is generally progressive, thus short-term. A few years ago the five-year fatality rate after a defining opportunistic infection was eighty-five percent. With medical progress, AIDS is evolving into a chronic, manageable disease, like diabetes, but this may not happen for the same five years, or for ten years, or for more. It's hard for me to write about AIDS: It's difficult to face yourself, confront your worst fears. I'm by nature a cynic, a pessimist. On the other hand, it's cheaper than therapy. On the (third?) hand, my former therapist died last year; I need not specify of what. It's also difficult to write about sex. Sex is a very private act. A certain part of me doesn't want to reveal everything, the frailties contained in the sexual act. But the best writing for me confronts the most difficult issues. Being a New York creature, I thrive on stress.

My editor has given me complete support in writing about sex and writing about HIV—although he decided against including "Queer and Loathing at the FDA" in *Spontaneous Combustion* because he felt it would confuse people into thinking that my writing wasn't fiction at all. Books dealing with HIV/AIDS aren't going to sell like Danielle Steel, but neither are books with primarily gay content. I write about sex and sexuality in a safe context as most do—even Dennis Cooper's ritual disembowelment scenes don't involve HIV transmission. My aim is to reflect experiences of being HIV-positive and gay life so people can recognize their feelings and feel less isolated.

There are an estimated 1.5 million HIV-positive individuals in the U.S. This estimate hasn't changed over the past few years. I guess we can all stop demonstrating and go home now: The epidemic is over, according to the government. But I have a sneaking suspicion that things will continue to get worse before they get better. I feel compelled to testify. I will continue to write about AIDS as long as I am able to because, in a sense, there really is no other topic.

I wrote this piece for a panel at the second OutWrite conference for gay and lesbian writers in 1991 in San Francisco. I was placed on a panel called "Writing and Disability." I felt somewhat illegitimate. Allan Barnett was offered my spot first; he declined, and proceeded to give a painful and maudlin paper on the difficulties of writing with AIDS for a fiction-writing panel. (He died on August 14, 1991.) I didn't have access to a personal computer: I was on vacation in San Francisco and hadn't finished this paper when I left New York. Consequently, it was handwritten. I had no idea how long it would take to read. At the conclusion of the panel, a lesbian complimented me on it, then proceeded to lecture me because the two men on our panel spoke for twice as long as the women. Luckily for me, no one from the audience addressed me during the question-and-answer period of the panel discussion. I am terrified of impromptu questions. This piece appeared in a somewhat different form in NYQ. It served as my introduction to the magazine. I was somewhat reluctant to submit it, as NYQ had published a piece about AIDS and writing a few weeks earlier.

Tales
from the
Front

Another dateless Saturday night and I sit, dejected, on the couch. Sigh. It's only nine o'clock. The Sunday *New York Times* lies in disarray on the carpet. I have already thumbed my way through the Arts and Leisure section, hoping for a large facsimile of Cher suitable for framing. Nothing this week. Why don't they give us fags a ten-cent discount? We never bother with the Sports. It's straight into the trash on the corner, before we've even come home.

Well, I *could* be adventurous and take a nap and wake up to the dissonant alarm at midnight and cab down to the Spike and spend a few hours looking bored drinking overpriced club sodas and then return home at four with a bloated bladder and a distended prostate. Or I could simply lift the receiver and dial 550-TOOL. Last month's phone bill was only eighty dollars.

It takes only a moment to decide.

Thanks to the miracle of phone sex, the man of my dreams (5′9″, 155 lbs., salt-and-pepper hair, thirty-eight, hard muscular build) is on his way to my apartment. He should arrive in less

Originally appeared in Diseased Pariah News, *Issue 2, Spring 1991.*

than half an hour. I decide to wait to tell him my seropositive status until after my latex-wrapped pulsating manhood is twelve inches deep into his tight-gripping love canal. Okay, so maybe I'm lying. Who cares, so long as we have antiseptic safe sex.

Fuck. I haven't shaved in several days. My face feels like sandpaper. Maybe my Dream Lover isn't into dermabrasion. I go into the bathroom and lather up.

Quick. He should be here in fifteen minutes. I take a few cautious strokes, then glide my way through the cream like a hot knife through butter. A red maraschino-cherry blot appears at the whipped cream of my chin. I cut my chin. I begin bleeding profusely. What am I, related to some Russain czarina? "Clot, dammit!" I swear to myself. HIV-infected blood pools into the basin. More gushing than blushing beauty, I stick on a Band-Aid, apply pressure.

A little shaving cream on my ear. Gently, I take my washcloth to wipe it off, knocking my earring into the sink. Of course it teeters to the trap of the drain. Where are my tweezers? I have none. Unfortunately, I am no drag queen manqué. The time I painted my nails red for Halloween, I had not had the necessary foresight to obtain nail-polish remover beforehand. The following morning, sheepish, hands in pockets, I went to the A&P for this compulsory cosmetic. And of course, the gentleman behind me asked that most insulting question: "Are you an actor?"

This is the second stud I lose. I had gotten my ear pierced a scant month ago at the imbecilic age of thirty-three, slow learner that I am. A Bart Simpson earring that I found at a Hallmark cardshop inspired me. Bart Simpson seems inappropriate for sex. I try to insert another earring, a tiny hoop. My sinistral ear starts bleeding.

I take off the Band-Aid on the chin. How can anyone possibly have sex with a Band-Aid on the chin? Once again begins the flow. Two Band-Aids later I find myself still a fount of blood.

What am I to do? Awash in a sea of infection and disaffection, mired in anxiety and despair, dropping T-cells by the minute, I sit and stare at my ghastly reflection in the mirror, pray for coagulation. Studmeister is on his way in a cab, ready for action. I'm locked in the bathroom, crying over my dowry of diseased precious bodily fluids.

Of course, he never shows. I don't have his number. He doesn't call with explanations.

Evidently, Some Higher Power is teaching me a lesson.

Why do I even bother with the phone-sex line? I'm bound to be disappointed. Even if Mister Wrong showed up and was as appealing as he indicated, what would be the likelihood of sustaining a relationship that would last five minutes past orgasm? Surely I have experienced enough personal growth that I don't need to rely on cheap anonymous sex for kicks. How many more nights am I destined to wait fruitlessly in my humble abode for the Falcon video equivalent of Elijah? He'll never come. I'll never come. What's the point?

Two hours later, when the bleeding has finally subsided, I dial that elusive number again. This time, I go to *his* place.

••

I love Diseased Pariah News, *a 'zine by and for the HIV-infected that comes out of San Francisco whose motto is "No Teddy bears." I was delighted to make it into the second issue with this piece. Black humor reigns at DPN. When one of the first editors died, Beowulf Thorne (not the name he was born with), the surviving founding editor, mixed some of his ashes into the ink. Beowulf is the creator of the comic strip "Captain Condom." In a recent issue of DPN, Captain Condom gets thrown into jail for beating up Louise Hay. Need I say more?*

I eventually had to place a block on my phone. My compulsive phone sex combined with a sticky call-waiting button was bound to lead to an embarrassing conversation with a close blood relative. Of course, I imme-

diately found a loophole involving credit cards. But now, in my new apartment, the phone is on the desk and the bed is miles away. Phone sex is no longer . . . convenient. I know, I could always get a longer cord. It just doesn't seem worth the effort.

Direct Mail
From Hell

Back in the early sixties, there was an appalling show called "Queen for a Day." Contrary to your expectations, it wasn't the biography of Cobra Woman Maria Montez or an ongoing series on female impersonators. Four women would tell their pathetic tales of woe to the studio audience: how Hubby drank his way out of work and his mother lived upstairs in an iron lung and the house burned down when Junior tried to make a tuna-noodle casserole in the oven and neglected to light the pilot until it was too late and how it would be really nice if she could get a Maytag washer-dryer because it's really quite arduous beating the sheets on the rock down by the stream and doing laundry for twelve. Then the audience got to vote on the patented Applause Meter who was the most pathetic. The winner was crowned with an ersatz tiara and loaned an ermine wrap and taken to her dream kitchen. The losers got cents-off coupons at Safeway.

Well, at the end of the month when I sit at the kitchen table, sorting out the fund-raising mail I received in the past four weeks,

Originally appeared in NYQ, *February 23, 1992.*

sometimes I feel like a member of the audience of "Queen for a Day." With stern posture I pore over plaintive pleas for checks or charge-card authorizations ("Please Do Not Send Cash in the Mail"), the director at open auditions for the bus-and-truck-company version of *Death of a Salesman*. Who shall live and who shall die? Another sip of Chablis and I continue.

Mother Hale sends me a paperback about Hale House written by her daughter, which goes straight into the recycling bin. Mothers Against Drunk Driving have printed up return-address labels for me with only one minor typo. AmFAR includes a personally licked stamp on the return envelope, which is too difficult to steam. GMHC is like an overly attentive boyfriend, with weekly reminders and progress reports on the AIDS Walk and Dance-A-Thon; sometimes I wonder whether eighty percent of the money I may raise will be spent on our "relationship." I got at least seven copies of last year's ACT UP acquisitional fund-raiser: Luckily for me, they had weeded out duplicates; if not, I'm sure I would have received twenty-seven. I wonder whether by not checking the box to ensure that my name won't be traded I'm inadvertently killing rain forests. Several of my gay male friends, all in their early thirties, regularly receive postcards from Trinity Memorial, advertising cemetery monuments and funeral plots. Did they steal Wonder Bar's mailing list? "Your first-class stamp will help us save money," claims the envelope, with "No postage necessary if mailed in the United States" printed where a stamp would be affixed. Conflicting signals. The year-end fund-raising letter I receive on December 30 is almost immediately followed by the plea to renew my annual support on January 2.

I used to get so excited knowing that Elizabeth Taylor, Harvey Fierstein, and Mary Tyler Moore were writing to me personally. Alas! There is no tooth fairy! And everybody knows that professional fund-raisers write the letters, not the signatories. I found this out when a candidate for public office who coincidentally ran a direct-mail operation sent out fund-raising letters that were almost identical to ACT UP fund-raisers using the signature of an activist who hadn't even read the letter.

So what I do is ignore the letters, stuff the perforated forms into the return envelopes, and periodically go through them, maybe once a month. My cousin has MS, so I'll send them something. Everybody supports cancer research: Why should I? Conversely, I try to support every AIDS organization I find, because I really don't think they're that "popular" in terms of charities. I can justify not working in an AIDS-related field by donating money to AIDS organizations. I'd probably completely burn out if I worked for one. Let's face it, some days I'm sick of AIDS. Can't we go to the movies instead?

But occasionally the letters will be so appalling that I have to respond.

I recently received two letters so atrocious that I was compelled to write to the senders. I'm still not sure which was the more odious. The Los Angeles Shanti Project sent me a mailing with the note ". . . AIDS has improved the quality of my life . . ." in 30-point lavender on the envelope. The temptation to California-bash was irresistible: Anything would improve the quality of life in that cultural wasteland, wouldn't it? The enclosed letter was thoughtfully printed in large type for the visually impaired. It was the usual shit about achieving some *fuller understanding* of life and love. For some reason, as an HIV-positive person, I didn't get it. I'm just dense, I guess. I know, there's a silver lining in every cloud and a Louise Hay ready to make an economic killing finding it, and I thank God every day that She chose me to be sacrificed for the sins of the heteros, and as I'm rotting on the cross of CMV retinitis and pneumocystis and toxoplasmosis and a host of other viral and bacterial infections and dementia strikes, I'll still consider myself lucky. Not! I really find such asinine shock tactics as using the pathetically misguided quote ". . . AIDS has improved the quality of my life . . ." extremely offensive. But, then again, I'm a cynical

New Yorker with virtually no inner life. It could be *my* problem.

The second, closer to home, was from Lambda Legal Defense and Education Fund. On the envelope, scrawled in messy cursive next to my address, was the phrase "Before he died, he asked me to mail this to you." It was from Bob Bradley, brother of the teacher from Long Island who sued Blue Cross to pay for a bone-marrow transplant that he was ultimately unable to undergo because he developed CMV during the settling of the suit. I really appreciate the thought that on his deathbed, when most people are worrying about the afterlife, having religious conversions, cutting people out of their wills, reconciling with family members, or arguing with ex-lovers, Tom Bradley summoned his last bit of strength to dictate this letter and said to send it to me, DAVID FEINBERG, personally. He even thought to specify window envelopes. He even knew my ZIP+4! I thought *Death on the Installment Plan* was a French novel, not the latest fund-raising tactic. I thought that *Letter from a Dead Man* was some obscure Joan Crawford movie from the late forties. I thought that Lambda would have a little more style than to try to raise money from the corpses of dead PWAs. Why does it read as exploitation and tapping into "survivor's guilt" to me? Have they no shame?

One day I'll receive a letter that starts, "Hi, you don't know me, but I'm dead. I died of AIDS, and indeed, this greatly improved the quality of my life. I now reside in Queens at a beautiful cemetery overlooking the East River, and could you please donate $100 to pay for my monument?" And at the bottom of the page there'll be this note "over," and I won't turn the page.

••

Someone from Lambda called me to apologize. He blamed an outside consultant for this appeal. It turns out that the claim was literally correct. A year earlier, Tom had authorized a fund-raising appeal. It was so successful that Lambda decided to send it again. In the interim, Tom had died.

The Shanti Project chose to ignore my complaint. A week later I ran into a tall and slender beauty with only three visible flaws at my gym who admitted culpability. The direct-marketing company he worked for was responsible for Shanti's letter. He said that he felt the letter accurately reflected the organization. Needless to say, I have been dropped from that particular mailing list.

Sex Tips
for Boys

Or, What to Do When the Guy You Met in the Steam Room Wants to Get to Know You Better before He Lets You Put His Penis in Your Mouth; Or, Dates from Hell

Recently, I've had an unrelenting stream of bad dates. Indeed, were it not for my shining knight in Montreal whom I met at a bathhouse so sleazy that the dryer was broken and consequently patrons were given wet towels, I believe I would have completely lost hope in all humanity, or at least that portion of humanity with which I might possibly get laid. For some reason, nobody wants to have sex with me these days, save that occasional bulimic Adult-Child-of-Alcoholics novelty dancer who keeps calling me at odd hours. There *was* a rather enjoyable hour of foreplay *interruptus* in the hotel room of an extremely attentive young man last week, but then again, he was from L.A., which more or less negates any possibility of consummating the deed in the future, near or distant. Before that was the cute but unfortunately overly introspective neuropsychiatric resident whose ex-lover was dying of leukemia who told me that he was initially drawn to me because of his subliminal death wish and perhaps given my serostatus I could be an agent of his death, whereas I in fact preferred to be known as an instrument. And before that was the gentleman (al-

Originally appeared in QW, *May 17, 1992.*

though perhaps it would be a stretch to refer to him using this descriptive, since douche-bag would be more appropriate) whom I picked up at the gym, had sloppy and not particularly memorable sex with, and then two weeks later to the day when I saw him at the gym as I was doing forty-pound curls had the following conversation with:

"Hi, Mike."

Genially: "Hi." Pause.

(Figuring he'd forgotten my name) "It's Dave."

"Oh." Bigger pause. "I know I know you from somewhere. I'm sorry, but I just can't place it."

Huge pause. "The gym."

Quick beat. "Oh, yeah. You came over that evening."

Brief pause. "It must be my new haircut." The one that looks identical to my previous 'do.

Of course, what I should have said was, "It's quite understandable that you wouldn't remember me because, being a clone, I look exactly like the last fifteen men you've had sex with, whereas your quite distinct acne scars make you what Natalie King Cole sang last year in the necro-incest duet with her dead father, *unforgettable*."

But now everyone I meet wants to have *relationships*. I refer specifically to the failed actor I met last month under extremely tawdry circumstances at my gymnasium whose testicles I have, in fact, felt in the palm of my hand, as if I were comparison-shopping for produce at the local A&P. Quite exquisite, I might add. Well, Walter (not his real name) decided that he wanted to get to know me better before we did the nasty. Gleefully, I referred him to the local bookstore, thinking that perhaps he could purchase and read both of my admittedly autobiographical novels. Since he felt a need to get to know me better and I didn't necessarily feel the same need, I didn't understand why I had to be physically present as he "got to know" me. Nonetheless, I proceeded to undergo a series of quite enjoyable (and to my mind, quite beside the point) dinners and movies and the occasional shopping expedition with him: I believe they're known as "dates" in common parlance. Still no nookie. "Walter" still felt that I was primarily interested in having sex, and the only reason that he was the object of my interest was physical proximity. Frankly, I didn't understand how we could have sex otherwise.

I decided to do what I usually do, which is make a list, comparing reasons to sleep with someone immediately and reasons not to:

Reasons Not to Sleep with Someone Immediately
1.

I decided that I would write the second list first, and by the time I finished the second list, perhaps one or two reasons to wait would spontaneously occur to me.

Reasons to Sleep with Someone Immediately
1. Your combined T-cells taken as SAT scores wouldn't get either of you into the tiniest, most decrepit community college in the state of Iowa, and they have open admissions there.

2. To know, know, know you is *not* necessarily to love, love, love you. As a matter of fact, the more appropriate proverb here is "familiarity breeds contempt."

3. "I'd love to blow you but I just did pentamidine" doesn't really cut it as a good excuse. Why else did God invent breath mints and peppermint-swirled candies?

4. Just because he suffered the humiliation of having his braces entangled when he kissed his second cousin Matilda when he was fourteen, there is no reason to repeat the trauma at thirty-five by getting his IV entangled with yours at some future date. *Carpe frenulum!* Seize the Dick!

5. Sexual intercourse can be an extremely intimate form of nonverbal communication. If he really wants to know you better, what better way than by fornication? Indeed, sex can function as an excellent "ice breaker" in terms of breaking down barriers and thus facilitating future intimacy. On the other hand, if he wishes to keep his distance, there is a multitude of ways to have sex that would not necessarily impinge on anyone's personal space.

With Jeffrey Dahmer in prison and Roy Cohn most decidedly dead, I still haven't come up with any adequate reasons not to sleep with someone on the first date. I suppose there's always that character issue. You could fall asleep next to some gorgeous hunk and wake up next to a design professional or, worse yet, an actor. But, hey, why be picky? Discrimination is against the law. Moreover, it's tacky. If anyone knows of any good reasons to wait, please let me know. You know where to find me.

••

I alienated at least three people with this piece. I wrote it for Diseased Pariah News, *but because of* DPN's *backlog, it was eventually published in* QW.

AIDS
and
Humor

If art is to confront AIDS more honestly than the media have done, it must begin in tact, avoid humor, and end in anger.

Avoid humor, because humor seems grotesquely inappropriate to the occasion. Humor puts the public (indifferent when not uneasy) on cozy terms with what is an unspeakable scandal: death. Humor domesticates terror, lays to rest misgivings that should be intensified. Humor suggests that AIDS is just another calamity to befall Mother Camp, whereas in truth AIDS is not one more item in a sequence, but a rupture in meaning itself. Humor, like melodrama, is an assertion of bourgeois values; it falsely suggests that AIDS is all in the family. Baudelaire reminded us that the wise man laughs only with fear and trembling.

—Edmund White, "Esthetics and Loss,"
Artforum, January 1987

Delivered as a talk at OutWrite on March 20, 1992; published as "Is Humor an Acceptable Way to Deal with AIDS?" in The Advocate, *Issue 609, August 13, 1992.*

Well, it's a beautiful argument. I don't know about you, but I was convinced, at least for the moment. Good writing can persuade one of almost anything. Extraordinary how potent cheap logic is.

At the same time, the argument is completely vacuous. Out of context, the statement "AIDS is a rupture of meaning" is so ludicrous it's almost funny, a beautiful phrase, but itself an absurd rupture of logic, or perhaps symptomatic of a beleaguered author's cerebral hemorrhage.

That's the trouble with pontifications from *Artforum* and the like. Grand pronouncements are good for rhetorical discussions and little else. If you're clever enough, you can easily come up with just as convincing an argument on the opposing side of the issue. Save it for the high-school debate team.

It's completely unnecessary to demolish his arguments point by point. I need only mention several examples of the successful use of humor in art about AIDS: William Hoffman's play *As Is;* Paul Monette's novels *Afterlife* and *Halfway Home*; Peter McGehee's novel *Boys like Us*; Christopher Durang's monologue about AIDS in *Laughing Wild*; *Diseased Pariah News*; John Weir's *The Irreversible Decline of Eddie Socket*; Victor Bumbalo's play *Adam and the Experts*; Matias Viegener's story "Twilight of the Gods"; and my novels, *Eighty-Sixed* and *Spontaneous Combustion*. Indeed, it is hard to find any work that does not at least deal with humor peripherally, save the sober sanctimonious holier-than-thou *Death Be Not Proud* school of humorless literal-minded writing.

I read *Death Be Not Proud* in high school and loathed it. I couldn't stand this flawless paragon with a brain tumor. I felt as if I were trapped at a six-hour testimonial dinner on an ocean liner. The poor kid was merely a composite of every good trait imaginable: He ceased to be an individual.

I'm not going to produce a pretentious series of implacable dictims and Rules One Must Follow if one is to write about AIDS with humor. I'm not going to hand out lofty precepts from this lectern like "Ensure that you include a partially abled ovolactovegetarian lesbian of color in a prominent position in your work not as tokenism but as affirmative action" or "All writing must deal with the AIDS crisis in an ethical fashion, and all other writing, such as the ritual disembowelments of a certain perennial Lambda Literary Award nominee, is inherently decadent and morally corrupt."

My goal here is to simultaneously demystify and obfuscate, two words I swore I would never use in polite company. Just kidding. There are no rules. You do whatever you can. You do whatever works. Instead, I'm going to suggest several ways that humor might be effectively used in writing about AIDS.

Consider the centrality of humor in everyday life. People are constantly making jokes. Waitresses wisecrack as they pour you a cup of java; the four hunky window washers whom you secretly envision in some porno scenario are in fact joking about the clutter in your office and secretly redesigning it; girlfriends dish one another at the gym; your mother complains about the fact you haven't called in a million years with an amusing twist of irony; your boyfriend offers to play "Hide the Sausage" with you; it goes on and on.

Nothing is off limits to humor, not even the Holocaust. I recall the scene in Paul Mazursky's movie *Enemies*, when Angelica Huston announces to Ron Silver, "I'm dead." Mel Brooks wrote a movie that centered on a surprise hit play called *Springtime for Hitler*. Perhaps the only time the limits of taste were breached in the past twenty years was with the television sit-com "Hogan's Heroes," which took place in a German prisoner-of-war camp during World War II.

Joseph Heller's masterpiece about war, *Catch-22*, is perhaps the best example I know of black humor. Heller comments on the absurdity of life during wartime with a deadpan voice. He achieves his great effect at the climax by juxtaposing humor with tragedy. The reader is softened for the kill with jokes; at the end, no punches are pulled. This contrast can achieve a great emotional impact.

In an absurd world, humor may be the only appropriate response. I used a quote from Barthes as an epigraph to *Eighty-Sixed*: "What I claim is to live to the full the contradiction of my time, which may well make sarcasm the condition of truth."

Humor is a survival tactic, a defense mechanism, a way of lessening the horror. I would probably literally go mad if I tried to deal with AIDS at face value, without the filter of humor.

Once you joke about something, you appropriate it, you attain a certain amount of control over it. For example: "My T-cells recently dropped below my IQ. It's a good thing I'm not Amy Hempel, or I'd be legally dead."

Humor is also used as a distancing medium: You can't stare directly at the sun. When someone asks, "How can you be so flip?," I respond, "How can you not be?"

There's always that ever-popular gallows humor. I've occasionally played a game of trying to think of extremely inappropriate songs to be played at one's memorial: Maureen (Queen of Disaster Movies) McGovern's "There's Got to Be a Morning After," Marilyn McCoo's "One Less Bell to Answer," and Peggy Lee's immortal "Is That All There Is?" come to mind.

Noël Coward wrote: "Extraordinary how potent cheap music is." I've always had a weak spot for cheap humor: the silly pun, the bad joke.

Joni Mitchell, that great Canadian sage of our time, equates laughter and crying as methods of emotional release in her classic "People's Parties," one of those favorite songs I used to listen to when I was an adolescent girl in Syracuse, New York. It has been suggested that perhaps I still am that same adolescent girl. In any event, faced with the AIDS crisis, sometimes one laughs to avoid crying.

I'm interested in the joke that makes you wince as you laugh or suppress a smile; the joke that simultaneously appeals and appalls;

the joke on the edge; the uncomfortable joke; the joke that catches you unaware, where your first response is to laugh and you immediately check yourself, ashamed.

Some may say that only HIV-positive writers can deal with AIDS, and they are beyond criticism. How can someone personally unaffected by the epidemic accuse a writer with AIDS of acting inappropriately, disrespectfully, and without dignity? This argument is absurd. As if identity can authenticate work. Gary Trudeau's "Doonesbury" episodes show one doesn't have to be seropositive to write about AIDS with humor.

Humor is extremely subjective. If it misfires, it can be deadly. Of course, everything I've said will sound ludicrous and hopelessly pompous to someone who doesn't "appreciate" my sense of humor, and I use the word *appreciate* guardedly; I mean someone who has similar tastes in humor as I have. Failed humor trivializes tragedy and offends the reader, as I'm sure I've offended many.

When the humor doesn't work for you, consider the moral intent of the writer. AIDS jokes are generally repugnant because the intent is to poke fun at people with AIDS. A few years ago, I read a novel with an AIDS theme and it rang patently false to me. I couldn't quite put my finger on what I didn't like about it until someone told me that the author wrote it hoping it would be turned into a disease-of-the-week movie. If you dislike a work, consider what the author's intent was: Did the author try to share experiences and use humor to get closer to the bitter truth, or was the humor merely added to be outrageous? Before you completely dismiss a work as bankrupt, consider the underlying intent. This is not how you judge a work on literary merit, but how you can forgive one for failing.

••

I wrote this for the third OutWrite conference in Boston, 1992. I was on a panel with John Weir, Victor Bumbalo, and Matias Viegener. Larry Kramer spent the conference disrupting the Q & A portions of the sessions

with pointed questions, and then storming out angrily. "Can anyone explain irony to me?" was his pointed question. Unfortunately, we all tried
but failed.

I've been called the Henny Youngman of AIDS by a columnist in that
most esteemed publication, the New York Native, but that was by the
same person who referred to my best friend in the entire world, John Weir,
as "the late John Weir" in another column. John, who is very much alive,
was inspired to write a letter to the editor to the effect that reports of his
early demise were gross exaggerations. Following is an excerpt from his letter (New York Native, *August 24, 1992*):

> Then an unnerving thing happened. We were strolling past the
> Chelsea Hotel, when an old friend of mine walked out of the lobby
> and shrieked. "What are you doing here?" he said. I admitted that
> I still got north of Fourteenth Street, occasionally, shocking as that
> sounded. "No," said my friend, "I mean, what are you doing on
> the planet? I thought you were dead."
>
> In fact, I had assumed that he was dead, too, since I hadn't seen
> or heard from him in about two weeks.
>
> "I'm still here," I said, reassuring him.
>
> My friend looked disappointed. "Now I'll have to put you back
> in my Rolodex," he said, disgruntled.

The letter was signed "John Weir, Still alive and well and living on
East Eleventh Street." The editors responded, "The Native *apologizes
for this embarrassing error.*"

April
Fools

I'm getting AIDS this Wednesday, April 1, at 12:01 A.M. This is
not to say that I am destined to reach a critical point in terms of
the mathematical growth of infected cells in my lungs at midnight;
this is not because I can pinpoint the precise moment when I was
infected with HIV (August 17, 1982, at approximately 1:47 in the
morning in some seedy establishment best left to the imagination), and it is statistically inevitable that I come down with a defining disease exactly nine years, seven months, thirteen days,
twenty-two hours, and fourteen minutes after initial exposure because I have consciously striven to be Joe Clone (the average gay
man, virtually indistinguishable from anyone else) for the past
decade and therefore I am the statistical mean.

I'm getting AIDS this Wednesday, April 1, at 12:01 A.M. because my T-cells have consistently been under 200 for the past
year and the Centers for Disease Control's definition of AIDS is
scheduled to change on April 1 to include, in addition to a rather
long list of opportunistic infections and diseases, the fewer-
than-200 T-cell criteria. April fool! I've got AIDS. The CDC

Originally appeared as "Getting AIDS Absurd" in NYQ, *April 5, 1992.*

definition was supposed to change on January 1. I was dreading New Year's Eve for all the usual reasons (the strictly enforced gaiety of the season, the inability to consume vast quantities of alcohol without forcibly vomiting two hours later, and, most important, physical proximity to Times Square); in addition, I was dreading it because I was going to get AIDS. And now it probably looks as if the definition will not change for another few months (but maybe it will). The CDC announced the prospective definition last fall and has been extending the comment period and changing the effective date due to pressure from activists, community-based organizations, physicians, and me, mainly because I don't want to get AIDS.

Last year I blithely assumed that the Immigration and Naturalization Service would completely open the borders to people with HIV on June 1 for the absurd reason that it said it would; however, in response to massive pressure from right-wing conservatives, it softened the regulations so people with HIV could visit but not stay in the U.S. Which is why the international AIDS conference was moved to Amsterdam. Frankly, I think this was a cynical move on behalf of the government to bankrupt ACT UP/N.Y., which plans on sending more people to Amsterdam than the entire Division of AIDS (although theoretically it shouldn't [appreciably] cost ACT UP/N.Y. that much because the working group is committed to raising 95 percent of the money itself, and has indeed already raised 1.3 percent).

On April 1 I am scheduled to move from asymptomatic HIV-positive to the absurd and oxymoronic appellation *asymptomatic AIDS*. I feel unworthy of this transition; this is an undeserved honor for me. I feel I should go through some rite of passage first. I'm not ready for the psychological jet lag of this nomenclatural change, a purely numerical boundary that leaves me with the nauseating vertigo one gets from switching ZIP codes at a dizzying rate. I much prefer the comfort of traveling by train. It is as if I could get to heaven without dying.

This is just another anxiety reaction I'm going through. I spent the entire year I was twenty-nine dreading thirty. After surviving my birthday, my anxiety completely dissipated. Now the tables are turned and my three main goals in life are to find a lover, to travel to Italy, and to live to forty (not in that order). So it's conceivable that after April 1 I will no longer wake up at 6:00 A.M. on Monday morning (for some reason every morning seems to be a Monday) with that dark feeling in my gut that is either total and absolute fear or indigestion.

I have three options to avoid getting AIDS on April 1. I could meditate and stop eating red meat and stick myself with needles and completely change my lifestyle to eliminate all anxiety, hence raise my T-cells above 200. The easier way out would simply be to stop time by bombing the international clock in Greenwich, England. Or I can resume my long-lapsed subscription to the *New York Native*, that Never-Never Land where "AIDS" doesn't exist except as a construct in quotes.

What should I do when I come down with CDC-defined asymptomatic AIDS? Should I quit my job to devote my time to writing, which may in fact be no longer possible given the unlimited time and lack of distraction? I cannot comprehend how anyone could face the empty screen full-time. Should I throw a party at some unsuitable venue, like the historic site of the Mineshaft, to which, oddly enough, I have never been?

My main concern is how I can work this to my advantage. Are there ways to exploit the system that has already exploited me beyond all reason? Can I get reduced-price tickets to the next Saint-at-Large party based on reduced T-cells? Is there a disability rebate through the phone company for certain grossly expensive exchanges? Will public assistance pay for poppers?

A major problem with the proposed definition is that gynecological manifestations of AIDS are not addressed in an adequate fashion. As I adopt my most paternalistic tone of male privilege, I state these poor beleaguered women with pelvic inflammatory disease and chronic vaginal candidiasis should be thankful that they won't be saddled with the additional stigma of having AIDS while I shall have to suffer this undeserved diagnosis. Who needs health care when we have cranberry juice? Readers of *NYQ* already know about the pitfalls of the proposed definition from previous articles by members of ACT UP/N.Y.'s CDC working group (one of whom is coincidentally on the editorial board of *NYQ*, which may lead one to wonder whether the coverage of a recent demonstration by the CDC working group was balanced). Nonetheless, inspired by the somewhat controversial tactics of the CDC working group and my own increasing anxiety, I am planning to handcuff myself to my own personal health-care practitioner on April 2 until the end of the AIDS crisis.

The proposed new definition still focuses on infections white gay men get, as opposed to intravenous-drug users, people of color, and women. Unfortunately, in the egocentric world I live in, I'm freaked. David B. Feinberg, This Is Your Life! Like *Jaws II*: This time it's personal. It took me two years to get used to being HIV-positive. I don't know if I'll have another two years to get used to having AIDS. Why can't we go back to that equally ridiculous construct, HIV disease? It's such a vague, amorphous term, not likely to attract dismal connotations simply because it is such a compound term. I suppose all terminology is problematic: "Homosexual" is a clinical mix of Greek and Latin affixes; "gay" is a unisyllabic male-leaning term absurdly conjoined with a nearly defunct adjective seemingly chosen at random; "fag" is an angry appropriation of a self-loathing epithet; "queer" is a gender-neutral term with perhaps even more self-loathing.

Several years ago, ACT UP had a demonstration at the National Institutes of Health. Members of ACT UP/N.Y.'s Treatment and Data Committee had placards that said "200 T-cells = AIDS." There was and still is an argument that by adding the 200 T-cell criterion to an already burgeoning list of diseases, one would be able, in one fell swoop, to cover all of those whose immune systems were sufficiently impaired. It didn't seem possible to keep up with all of the potential malfunctions of the immune system. It made sense to me at the time; but then again, I was in the 400 to 500 range. Although HIV test results are confidential in some states (but not others), there currently is no confidentiality anywhere when it comes to T-cell tests. T-cell tests are much more expensive than the HIV-antibody test. T-cell tests to be used effectively should be monitored over a period of time so that trends can be noted and T4/T8 cell ratios compared. People traditionally overlooked by the current definition—specifically, people without access to health care—will also be overlooked by the new T-cell-dependent criterion.

The real problem is that the official CDC definition of AIDS is used not just to diagnose AIDS, but to determine benefits. It's another political football. The science is sketchy and the research is incomplete. Health-care and disability benefits may depend on an AIDS diagnosis. I have friend who was constantly getting sick with minor ailments: He finally got his doctor to lie that he had thrush so he could get on Medicaid and disability. At this point in time, I would graciously offer to switch blood-test results with him (those lab-test mix-ups are common) if he needed additional certification.

But I'm left with the fact that I am probably going to get AIDS on, if not April 1, some other unspecified date. Yet nothing has changed. It's only a word. I want to scream. I prefer to be known as a PWLTC (Person With Lousy T-Cells) instead. Still, I'm terrified. These are absurd times. It's Wayne's World. We only live in it.

••

Ultimately, I didn't get my AIDS diagnosis until January 1, 1993. The CDC delayed enacting the new definition due to protests. It eventually added two gynecological manifestations to the list. Oddly enough, I feel that things began deteriorating for me in January.

Bleeding Gums
from Hell

My gums bleed.

Sometimes this happens when I brush my teeth with the vigor of a street cleaner's brushes gone mad. I remove the toothbrush from my mouth to rinse off the foamy Colgate and notice that the bristles are tinged pink. This I can handle. Worse is when this happens spontaneously. I bite into a McIntosh and see the lipstick imprint on the apple crater. I rush to check my lips for excess makeup in the bathroom mirror and then I remember I don't do drag.

I am hardly prepared to register myself as a personal site for religious pilgrimages. It's not as if I bleed only on days of holy saints and Good Friday.

I'm not particularly fond of any of my bodily fluids.

I always carry a portable battery-operated liquid Dustbuster to instantly mop off those unsightly semen spills from the masturbatory bedsheets or the stomach of the occasional boudoir visitor. I pick at a wart on my index finger and five minutes later have stuffed my hand in a blood-soaked pocket. If mucous contained HIV, I would probably kill myself. I have interminable postnasal drip: My Barbra Streisand imitation wouldn't be complete without it.

At times I feel my body has been transformed into a factory of infection, a vessel of virus. The wheels and cogs are constantly turning, manufacturing more toxins and poisons. My body is merely the host.

But now my greatest fear is deep-kissing a stranger, and as our tongues mingle, tasting rust, I abruptly excuse myself to dash to the bathroom to spit blood.

I follow the regulations promulgated at the Sixteenth Annual International Conference on HIV Risk Reduction: Before putting your mouth on any organ or orifice of a prospective ex-boyfriend, use mouthwash, skip the toothpaste, and, above all, don't floss.

My mother had bad teeth. She would floss constantly: after dinner in the kitchen, in the living room in front of "All in the Family." My father preferred a toothpick, which my mother felt was lower-class. She made him go to the bathroom to perform this vulgar act. I didn't understand the difference. I never use dental floss.

My primary methods of seduction rely upon the hands and the mouth. Hands are for physical contact of any sort, from brushing against a stranger's thigh to rubbing a gentleman's neck to slowly tracing his spine. My hands, alas, are wart-besotted. The mouth is used for a series of outrageous lies and unbelievable promises, exaggerated store-bought flattery mixed with home-grown cynicism. Lips can caress the lip of a bottle of Bud, anticipating other lips and other cylindrical objects of affection.

At its worst, my mouth is reduced to several dozen bloody Chiclets.

So for the longest time, these two items rested at the top of my personal to-do list:

1. Get Rid of Warts.
2. Stop Bleeding Gums.

• • •

I have a bad history with dentists.

I close my eyes in the dentist's chair. I'm Dustin Hoffman in *Marathon Man*. Laurence Olivier drills into my mouth without using anesthesia. "Is it safe?" he implores.

I didn't take a shower for two months after seeing *Psycho*. I didn't see a dentist for five years after seeing *Marathon Man*.

Then I saw *Little Shop of Horrors*, with Steve Martin as the sadistic dentist and Bill Murray as the masochistic patient. Thereafter I avoided professional dental hygiene for another two years.

When I was nine, I deliberately bit my dentist on the hand, just to see how he would react. He ratted on me to my mom. He happened to be my first cousin once removed.

I go through a period when I only see dentists named Jeffrey and only date oboists named Mark.

In a moment of extreme poor judgment, I comment to an attractive young man I had met at the sleazy Body Center about the ridiculous dental factory I passed on Bleecker Street that I deemed "Bitter Slime." In an unfortunate coincidence, Jeffrey C. happens to be employed at said Better Smiles: He is, in fact, one of the two dentists. Out of guilt and embarrassment, I immediately make an appointment and see him for several years.

A few years later, I ask my friend Glenn Person for a dental recommendation. He refers me to Jeffrey H. Glenn is in late-stage AIDS at that time. Jeffrey discreetly asks me if I have a similar condition. I tell him no.

We go to the same gym.

Jeff is competent and mildly boring as dentists go. He once tells me an amusing joke about a woman who is being simultaneously examined by him and another dental professional. "I've always wanted to have two men in my mouth," she says. But then Jeff retires and moves to Florida. Jeff dies of AIDS about a year later.

· · ·

Wayne refers me to his exceptionally cute dentist, Russell. Unfortunately, I never even meet him. My first visit consists of an hour's worth of X rays with a gaily Hispanic mildly sadistic hygienist named Nanette, who is expecting twins in August. Calipers are used to measure gaps at my gums. This experience is altogether unpleasant. I neglect to make an immediate follow-up appointment. The office is relocating to another floor in the building in a week. The receptionist forgets to schedule my next appointment. A month later, when I return to get my gums planed, Russell is out with a sprained back. Three months later he is dead. AIDS, again. Brenda, the mildly obese receptionist who was either a textbook fag hag in love with her homosexual boss, a sympathetic lesbian, or a former backup singer for an orotund Bette Midler, has disappeared; she is either pregnant or grief-stricken. She has been replaced by a thin-lipped harpy from Queens who wears tight earrings that pinch.

Am I turning into Kimberly Bergalis?
  I guess it's too late to sue the estates.

This is Kimberly Bergalis in Hell: Every morning she wakes up at 7:00 A.M. to a ringing phone. Groggily, she picks up the receiver to hear, "Miss Bergalis? This is Dr. Acer's receptionist. I'm calling to remind you that your dental procedure has been rescheduled for today at five."

A stalwart Irish boy with a firm grip grinds my gums down to size on subsequent visits. I spit the requisite mouthful of blood into the bowl, and watch it swirl down the drain, chased by running water.

Are there any lesbian dentists in the tri-state area?

· · ·

The hygienist instructs me on the Water Pik. I am to use it nightly with water on the highest setting, and then, once again, with a fluoride solution. After flossing with diligence. After brushing my teeth. After taking my nightly pills. What a drag. This will be the last thing I do every night, when I am completely exhausted. My nocturnal routine has been lengthened by a good ten minutes. Strictly speaking, I should use the Water Pik twice a day, but nobody expects that level of compliance.

For a few weeks the only time I bleed is when I Water Pik at night. I wonder whether I am ameliorating or exacerbating the situation.

For some reason I am acutely embarrassed by my Water Pik. It becomes another most intimate of acts that I hide from the public. There seems to be no discreet way to disappear into the bathroom and Water Pik while some winsome youth is arrayed on the couch in a variety of seductive poses, listening to Tchaikovsky on the Victrola. There is no background noise loud enough to cover it: My Water Pik sounds like a Hamilton mixer on the Pulverize setting for grinding up bones. The Water Pik becomes yet another reason for avoiding sleep-overs, another chain around my neck. My overnight bag now consists of a handful of pharmaceuticals and vitamins, my contact-lens case, my saline solution, my cleaning solution, my Water Pik, the two nozzles, and a bottle of Peridex oral rinse. There's barely room enough for an extra pair of underwear and socks.

I go to Montreal to visit my favorite French-Canadian over Memorial Day weekend 1992. Although I use the Water Pik in the kitchen, I still manage to keep up Gabriel's roommate, along with the entire neighborhood in a two-block radius.

The next time I visit the hygienist I ask if I have to bring the Water Pik with me on vacations. Could I skip a few days and simply floss hourly instead? I am worried about European electrical currents and whether Evian water would be suitable in France. Visiting my family in upstate New York is traumatic enough as is.

He is obviously in a bad mood. In the most patronizing tone he could possibly adopt, he says, "You're not doing this for me."

I am having a seventies midlife crisis: I've grown sideburns and I'm dating an aerobics instructor. Binky is six-two, with jet-black hair. He never wears underwear.

One night I achieve a major intimacy breakthrough. Binky stays over, and while he disinterestedly flips through last month's *Inteview* magazine, I Water Pik *in his presence*. Like most potential boyfriends, Binky has minor commitment problems. At five o'clock he can't commit as to whether or not he is coming in from Queens to see me that night at ten.

Binky's HIV-negative, so he can nurse me through sickness and woe and pull the plug when the time comes. We enjoy quiet nights at home together, just sitting in front of the television and watching "A Current Affair," a show I had never heard of before I met Binky.

I truly love Binky. He makes every night we sleep together seem like a vacation. It is true bliss to kiss him good-night and cuddle with him for a few minutes. Unfortunately, the waking hours aren't quite as blissful. Binky has a mind of his own. He doesn't get along with any of my friends. As time goes by, I find him to be extremely passive-aggressive. Just my luck to fall for someone whom I eventually discover I have nothing in common with.

For about a year I keep up with the nightly dental hygiene. I use the Water Pik five or six times a week. I allow myself a vacation every week, just as I allow myself to skip an arbitrary exercise when I go to the gym. Then, abruptly, I stop. I seem to have no ill effects. My gums have stopped bleeding. Astonished, I keep this secret to myself on my next visit to the dentist. I expect to be sharply remonstrated. Perhaps they will even rap my knuckles with a metal ruler. Instead, I am encouraged to keep up with whatever I've been doing.

Now I use my Water Pik only on those rare occasions when guilt has so overwhelmed my being that I find it necessary to ex-piate my sins.

Every day for the rest of my fucking life.

100 Ways
You Can
Fight the
AIDS
Crisis

1. Wear a red ribbon to show your support of people with AIDS.

2. Explain to people who assume that you're color-blind and wearing mismatched clothing the significance of the red ribbon.

3. Consider tying a red ribbon around the throat of your least-favorite politician (e.g., Jesse Helms) until his eyes bulge and he turns blue.

4. Use a condom every time.

5. Distribute condoms at your local high school.

6. When short of change, a condom is always welcome at the collection plate, especially for liberal theologians such as Cardinal O'Connor.

7. Write letters to your local congresspersons demanding they double the research budget of the National Institutes of Health.

8. Shoot Jesse Helms.

9. Send telegrams to your senators demanding they respond to the AIDS crisis.

Originally appeared in LIFEbeat concert fund-raiser program, June 8, 1992.

10. Spray-paint stenciled messages on the street in front of the White House reminding the President that the AIDS crisis is not over.

11. Lobby for universal health care.

12. Vote for the presidential candidate who will do the best job combating AIDS.

13. Get your mom, your dad, your ex-lover, your sister-in-law, your nephew, your aunt, and your high-school math teacher to vote for the presidential candidate who will do the best job combating AIDS.

14. Poison Jesse Helms.

15. Chain yourself to the gates of the White House until the President takes responsible action on the AIDS crisis.

16. Join the massive AIDS Unity March and Rally on July 14.

17. Clip and send obituaries of people who have died of HIV-related illnesses along with a personal note to Barbara Bush at the White House.

18. Be visible as HIV-positive. Don't hide in the closet!

19. Don't lie in obituaries.

20. Shut down an obstreperous federal organization for a day.

21. Block the entrance to a pharmaceuticals company that is charging exorbitant prices for life-saving drugs.

22. Make a panel for the AIDS Memorial Quilt.

23. Make sure that the President sees the Quilt this time, and not from a helicopter fly-over.

24. Demonstrate against the INS to open the borders for people with HIV.

25. French-kiss a person with AIDS today.

26. Stir soup for God's Love, We Deliver.

27. Volunteer to be a buddy at GMHC.

28. Answer the phones at the Minority Task Force on AIDS.

29. Garrote Jesse Helms.

30. Donate a computer to the Women and AIDS Resource Network.

31. Take minutes at the ACT UP meetings.

32. Form a needle-exchange group.

33. Phone-zap local legislators when heinous repressive legislation is being proposed.

34. Fight homophobia. Hug a queer today.

35. Lynch Jesse Helms.

36. Fight sexism. Join NOW. March in the next pro-choice demonstration in Washington.

37. Fight racism. Let your elected officials know it is unacceptable to play golf at a restricted club.

38. Call for full funding of the Ryan White CARE Act.

39. Visit a friend in the hospital.

40. Go to benefits for AIDS organizations.

41. Donate money to AIDS organizations.

42. Volunteer time at local AIDS organizations.

43. Date people who work at AIDS organizations, or at least take them out to lunch.

44. Hang an AIDS banner from a prominent location (a highway overpass, a tall building, a church steeple, Marky Mark's underwear).

45. Buy more of those sexy *Red, Hot and Blue!* T-shirts.

46. Disrupt a politician's speech, demanding a response to the AIDS crisis.

47. Eviscerate Jesse Helms.

48. Organize a Tupperware party and distribute condoms, fact sheets, and safer-sex information.

49. Interrupt a live-news broadcast with AIDS-specific information and demands for continued coverage of the AIDS epidemic.

50. Become knowledgeable about the crisis. Learn the science. You are your best expert.

51. Combat AIDS-phobia in the workplace.

52. Nuke Jesse Helms.

53. Remember your friends who've died of AIDS.

54. Volunteer at an HIV ward.

55. Be sex-positive.

56. Fight to get women, IV-drug users, and people of color into drug trials.

57. Send postcards to the CDC demanding that it expand the definition of AIDS to include gynecological manifestations.

58. Tie up a discriminatory insurance company's fax and phone lines for a day.

59. Eliminate Jesse Helms with extreme prejudice.

60. Get arrested at an AIDS demonstration.

61. Stage a massive die-in on the lawn of a repressive politician's home (say, Jesse Helms's, for example).

62. Cover a repressive politician's home (say, Jesse Helms's, for example) with a condom the size of the Goodyear blimp.

63. Understand AIDS as a medical and political crisis.

64. Listen to Larry Kramer.

65. Don't believe everything you hear.

66. Don't believe everything you read in the papers.

67. Fight against AIDS hysteria. Spitting at a police officer is not "assault with a deadly weapon."

68. Be compassionate. We are all innocent victims.

69. Demand that public officials address the burgeoning TB epidemic.

70. Lobby for increased drug-treatment slots.

71. Flay Jesse Helms alive.

72. Combat homelessness. Support housing, not shelters.

73. Donate furniture to Housing Works, AIDS Resource Center, and other AIDS organizations that house the homeless.

74. Join ACT UP.

75. Volunteer to be on a community constituent group to give input on trials run by the AIDS Clinical Trials Group.

76. Build a mock graveyard of tombstones of people who have died from the government's neglect of the AIDS crisis and place it in a prominent location.

77. Fill a casket with bloody bones and place it in a prominent location with AIDS-related messages.

78. Set up a table or hand out flyers in a local shopping mall, town square, or community center.

79. Wheat-paste attention-grabbing posters or flyers around your community.

80. Organize a teach-in on AIDS-related issues at a local school, YW/MCA, YW/MHA, PTA meeting, church, mosque, or synagogue.

81. Donate services for a fund-raiser. Perform your amateur-magician act; read palms; tell horoscopes; kiss strangers; perform acupuncture; swallow swords; recite humorous anecdotes; make huge batches of marshmallow treats.

82. Never share needles. Clean needles and works with bleach between uses.

83. Don't be afraid to date someone with AIDS.

84. Although I haven't gotten any symptoms yet, my T-cells are lousy enough to qualify whenever they get around to changing the goddamned definition.

85. I'm in the book.

86. Don't hide from AIDS. Go to plays and movies that deal with the crisis. Read books that address AIDS.

87. Rent an advertising billboard and let your community know that the AIDS crisis is not over.

88. Fight against quarantines of HIV-positive people.

89. Cuisinart Jesse Helms.

90. Share your knowledge with your friends.

91. Organize a postcard mail-in campaign to a local legislator asking him or her to lobby the President for national leadership in response to the AIDS crisis.

92. Write letters to the editor of your local newspaper, discussing AIDS-related issues.

93. Phone in to local radio talk-shows and discuss AIDS-related issues.

94. Ask your local library to prominently display books and literature on AIDS and AIDS-related issues.

95. Organize a massive demonstration in front of a local government building that will raise public awareness about AIDS-related issues and the lack of federal leadership in responding to the AIDS crisis.

96. Take over the offices of a local politician, insurance company, or drug manufacturer: Chain yourselves to a desk or doorway and refuse to leave until your demands have been met.

97. Kill Jesse Helms. And while you're at it, take care of William Dannemeyer.

98. Do something every day to fight the AIDS crisis: Write a letter, make a phone call, attend a benefit, sleep with a PWA, set yourself on fire on the steps of the White House as a gesture of anger at the President's shoddy response to the AIDS crisis, write a check, share a drinking glass, visit a friend in the hospital, etc.

99. Don't burn yourself out trying to do everything all at once. Take care of yourself.

100. Use your imagination.

••

My friend Jim Baggett asked me to contribute a list for a benefit program. LIFEbeat, a nonprofit AIDS fund-raising organization associated with the music industry, was kicking off with a concert by the Pet Shop Boys, one of my favorite groups. I gave him a list of ten, and he said that I could do better than that. Incorporating some suggestions developed for the Kennebunkport action, when six busloads of ACT UP members invaded President Bush's summer retreat on Labor Day in 1991, I was able to get up to around ninety. I simply interspersed ten ways to kill Jesse Helms: Think of it as filler. I was predictably excoriated in the press. A columnist at the New York Native who didn't attend the benefit chose to review the program. He chided me for the inappropriateness of attacking Jesse Helms, who had just undergone invasive cancer surgery. In earlier work, I had written against the Native's AIDS coverage.

I felt its editorial slant on AIDS was purely lunatic fringe and completely irresponsible to the gay and lesbian community. And now I had succeeded in achieving a level of ignominy so low that the Native *hated me more than Jesse Helms.*

Cocktails
from
Hell

Fidelity is difficult for me in friends, lovers, and drugs. That's why I'm so pleased that my current personal health-care practitioner has put me on an excitingly varied new regimen of antiretrovirals! Not merely combination therapy, where I repeatedly batter the human immunodeficiency virus with toxic drugs and hope I myself don't expire from the impact of these blows; not merely alternation therapy, where that squirmy little virus gets a barrage of one-two punches. No, I am now doing alternating combination therapy. One month of AZT and ddI, and the next month of AZT and ddC. Second verse, same as the first. Et cetera *ad* perpetuity, or until the side effects overwhelm me or they lose effectiveness, which they may already have, or until the next generation of antivirals comes of age or until the insurance runs out or until I get in touch with my inner child.

It's sort of like subscribing to Harry and David's Antiretroviral of the Month Club.

I had been taking AZT for more than two years. To be precise, I took my first pill of AZT at an ACT UP meeting on August 28,

Originally appeared in QW, *September 6, 1992.*

1989. The date is emblazoned in my memory only because I forced my fictional alter ego, B. J. Rosenthal, to take *his* first pill of AZT on the very same date under identical circumstances. Fearing the ravages of premature Alzheimer's and AIDS-related dementia, I find these mnemonic devices quite helpful. Embarrassingly, a few weeks ago at work I was compelled to leave my office for a brief period on an urgent mission: in search of the Luke Perry cover of *Vanity Fair*. In the interim, I forgot the door combination. I felt sheepish enough to call a co-worker from a pay phone on the street. He slyly gave me the wrong combination.

So let me state for the written record that I took my first pill of ddI on Monday morning, May 11, 1992, at approximately 6:45 A.M. Actually, I took my first *two* pills at 6:45 A.M. The drug ddI comes in 50 and 100 mg dosages, and my doctor advised 150 mg, twice a day, on an empty stomach. I had the script filled the previous Friday; I let it sit over the weekend. No sense in rushing into things. Fools (and Judy Davis) rush in Where Angels Fear to Tread. A friend in Dallas, Texas, who recently found he was seropositive, despite years of rigid precautions save the occasional unprotected blowjob without ejaculation, told me he was planning on canceling a trip the following Tuesday should his T-cells be low enough to warrant starting AZT, because he wanted to monitor his condition under his physician's care. I told him that he might as well go; he could always Federal Express the daily blood tests to Metpath. As if. Oh, well. These *are* stressful times.

So what is ddI like? Imagine a huge white SweetTart the consistency of Kaopectate (that "pleasant-tasting antidiarrheal"). See Figure A to the right, Actual Size. After you've finished this article and you've read the phone-sex ad on the obverse side, you may cut out the sample ddI pill (Actual Size) for your own personal glory hole.

You can either chew ddI or mix it with water. If you choose to chew it, you will experience a sensation not unlike licking a sex partner's underarm after he or she used an antiperspirant with aluminum chlorhydrate. I prefer mine with water. I took my second dose of ddI on Monday, May 11, at 9:00 P.M., at a meeting of the AIDS Coalition to Unleash Power, at Cooper Union. I had purchased for this eventuality an 11.2-ounce bottle of Evian water, no doubt in tribute to Madonna's memorable performance in *Truth or Dare*. For some unfathomable reason, the 50 mg pills are just as large as the 100 mg pills. I gingerly opened the bottle and prepared to gently drop my two horse pills down the cavernous mouth. Appallingly enough, the pills were too large to fit. I had to break them up into quarters before shoving them down the mouth of the Evian bottle. I was agitated. I agitated the bottle. I wondered whether there was a brand of bottled water with a wide enough mouth. I myself rarely have problems fitting large objects into my own mouth. I gulped down twelve ounces of a tart, cloudy liquid and considered the alternatives: Chinese herbs, drinking my own urine, or an uncertain and untimely death. Some residue lay at the bottom of the bottle, impossible to dislodge without creating another water-faucet cocktail. I discarded the remains in the nearest receptable.

Henceforth I took my ddI with one or two ounces of water. Less is more. I break the tablets into four or five pieces and then stir them with a teaspoon. My friend Tom used to use cocktail shakers. Perhaps I could host a party of blender drinks: blue whales, saltless strawberry margaritas, and ddI cocktails. Daniel mixed his ddI with orange juice because he couldn't stand the taste. After a long weekend in Montreal over Memorial Day, I decided New York water mixed better than Canadian water; it must be the mineral content. I considered buying a coffee grinder before remembering that I didn't drink coffee. Somehow, a mortar and pestle reminded me of high-school chemistry labs and a series of failed experiments: In tenth grade I must have copied my entire chemistry notebook from Robert Strauss, and I ended up with only a C.

So the tablets are large enough to require a matched set of steamer trunks on wheels, not a pillbox. I'll deal. It's the "on an empty stomach" part that's tricky. I used to do AZT on an empty stomach based on the advice of one of those fifteen thousand medical circulars I collect: It was either ACT UP's *Treatment and Data Digest* or the *PWA Newsline* or *The Body Positive* or the AmFAR directory or the John James biweekly or GMHC's *Treatment Issues* or Martin Delaney's Project Inform newsletter. But then Larry Waites, M.D., of *The Advocate* told me otherwise. I think it was he. Does it really matter? Probably not. In any event, I don't think I'm capable of taking another drug three times a day on an empty stomach along with ddI twice a day on an empty stomach when an empty stomach means you ingest nothing in the two hours before and one hour following, but drugs may not be ingested until two hours following because the ddI buffer would inhibit proper absorption of the other drug. Unless I wanted to do the Gandhi thing. But I doubt the political efficacy of an antiretroviral fast, even on the steps of the Capitol.

So I wake up at 6:35 in the morning and mix up a batch of ddI cocktail and use it as my gym fuel instead of a bottle of Carboload, which is really nothing more than overpriced sugar-water with artificial colors so vivid I hear they're experimenting with them for gastrointestinal exams instead of the radioactive shit they use now. And if that means I'm stuck going to the gym seven days a week, tough luck. Or I drink enough decaffeinated lemon-zinger iced tea the previous night to guarantee arising at an unearthly hour for a predawn piss, and then I grind up some ddI elixir before collapsing back in bed, my erection long since whizzed out. The evening dose is taken two hours after an early dinner. I try to avoid untimely snacks. One night I even skipped dinner because it conflicted with my drug schedule; another night, I simply skipped the drug.

"Why not take the ddI at nine A.M. and nine P.M.?" my doctor suggests. "That's when I take it," he casually remarks. I suppose a certain sense of camaraderie can be gained by the frank admission of a doctor that he is undergoing the same regimen as his patients, along with, I fear, the inevitable anxiety that one's doctor may not survive the course of one's own treatment. But, again, I heard about a local physician who didn't divulge his illness to his patients; they were shocked and completely unprepared when he died suddenly, of AIDS.

This is the easy month. I'm taking underground ddC with AZT. The New! Improved! ddC, available at the PWA Health Group, is a reasonably sized pill. Quality control is better: The government isn't likely to urge them to take it off the market due to variable dosage again. I could even get the official ddC through some expanded-access program because my T-cells suck. I've already progressed (without even realizing it until I read the fine print) in terms of AZT failure by dropping below 200.

Luckily, I haven't had any side effects with either drug. None of that nasty peripheral neuropathy or potentially fatal pancreatitis. I'd already tried the Old! Variably Dosed! ddC from the PWA Health Group last fall. Here's a simple mnemonic to remember my alphabet-soup cocktails: I'm *D*oing *D*rugs *I*ntermittently or *D*rinking *D*eadly *C*ocktails in the hopes of *A* *Z*illion *T*-cells.

Michael Callen was once quoted as saying that taking AZT was like shooting a mosquito with a nuclear warhead. Bombs away! The data aren't in on either combination. An exceptionally intelligent AIDS activist was reportedly against ddC approval simply because there were no convincing data, but then again, Mark's a blond. I know that's an irrational dismissal. I used to be politically correct. I've since regressed. I would even consider dating someone who: (a) was an aerobics instructor, (b) aspired to be an actor, and (c) didn't wear underwear. As a matter of fact, I've already given him my keys. But isn't life itself a crap shoot? If I'm forced to make a decision in a vacuum, I might as well take a deep breath and try it.

•••

This appeared in QW after an interminable delay. As expected, QW cut my joke about the phone-sex ad. After reading this piece, Bob Caviano, founder of LIFEbeat, paid me the ultimate compliment one day by telling Jim Baggett, "Miss Feinberg understands."

I am planning on starting a column in a major periodical with wide-spread circulation titled "Miss Feinberg Understands." People could write me about any problem, no matter how ludicrous. For example, a reader from Manhattan writes: "I recently fell in love with my stepdaughter, and now my ex-wife, whom I've broken up with but never actually got married to; actually, I've never even lived with her, we keep separate apartments on the opposite sides of Central Park; she is claiming that I molested her seven-year-old adopted daughter. I didn't mean this to happen; love knows no reason. However, my ex is threatening to drag me through the dirt and ruin my career. She just doesn't understand. Could you help me?" Or, a reader from Waco, Texas, writes: "I've always believed that in America one should be free to worship whomever one chooses. Also, I strongly support the principle that under the Constitution every American has a right to bear arms. There are some people from the Bureau of Alcohol, Tobacco, and Firearms who disagree. They just don't understand. What should I do?"

No matter what the problem, I would always have one stock reply: Miss Feinberg understands.

Bob Caviano died on September 22, 1992.

Larry Waites died of AIDS-related causes in the fall of 1993.

Nam Yoho Renge Kyo

I was walking up Seventh Avenue on my way to a fund-raiser when I came across Richard, a deranged poet who used to smoke too much dope but now chants instead. Richard was in the category of cute-possible-boy-toy-but-unfortunately-too-spacey-to-make-a-date-with. Richard decided to accompany me. I knew he wouldn't actually go to the fund-raiser because money was involved.

"Let me tell you a story, Dave. I want to get your reaction," said Richard.

"Fine."

"There were two lovers from San Francisco and they were both HIV-positive."

"Is this a joke?" I interrupted.

"No. This really happened. After they tested positive, they decided to chant. They chanted *nam yoho renge kyo* for three months. Then they got tested again, and guess what? They were negative."

I said, "Bullshit bullshit bullshit bullshit bullshit bullshit bullshit bullshit bullshit bullshit bullshit bullshit bullshit bullshit bullshit bullshit bullshit. Why are you telling me this bullshit?"

Richard replied, "Well, of course, if you didn't believe in it, it wouldn't work for you." And this is when I had my Joan Crawford moment. Usually, you think of a snappy response three days later in the shower or on the toilet or when you're stuck on the E train because there has been a police action at Forty-second Street and the train has been held indefinitely, but today everything was crystal clear; it was as if I were Joan Crawford, and some demented scriptwriter who had been up until five in the morning high on reds rushed to the set and handed me today's nasty dialogue just as I strode out of makeup wearing six-inch fuck-me pumps and an Adrian design with shoulders out to Cleveland.

"Are you HIV-positive?" I said, omitting his name because at that point I was so furious I couldn't recall it.

"No," responded Richard.

"Well, then maybe if you chant long and hard enough, you'll seroconvert, too."

A few days ago I saw a Person Without Permanent Housing outside the local ATM. A Smartly Dressed Woman with Matching Handbag and Shoes had just handed him a card, which I assumed was a referral for social services or shelter. But she didn't leave: She wanted to be sure that he understood the contents of her card. An act of altruism on Twenty-third Street. How nice, I muttered to myself. At her direction, he read the card aloud: *"Nam yoho renge kyo."*

Oddly enough, Richard didn't come to my reading later that week.

Needles
and Pins

For the most part, it's no big deal with me: It's just a tingly feeling in my hands and feet. You've felt it when your ex comes over at three in the morning hysterical because his new boyfriend dumped him and his therapist is on vacation and even though it took you three years and four therapists to get over him when he dumped you, you turn the cheek and comfort him, although not in a sexual manner because that would be far too dangerous, and then he inexplicably falls asleep with your left arm around his shoulder and you can't move your arm for fear of inadvertently waking him up because he has a tendency to shriek like a car siren and fall to pieces when awakened from a trauma-induced psychological coma and your neighbor across the hall will probably retaliate with all six compact discs of Barbra Streisand if this goes on for one more night and consequently your arm falls asleep. Once in a while it feels as if I'm walking on pins and needles that have been heated to 460°F and I've forgotten to deaden the nerves through the power of suggestion, but that usually doesn't last more than a minute. A few weeks ago (July 15, 1992, to be precise, according to my Dream Diary) I dreamed I was experiencing anal neuropathy: a tingly but not altogether unsatisfying feeling along

117

the posterior end of the alimentary canal, and I thought, Jesus, not *another* sexually transmitted disease, but then it turned out that my rude boyfriend was trying to fuck me in my sleep. One can speculate that it might be nice to have an occasional bout of penile neuropathy: Imagine a thousand tiny fingers urging you to let go with your own built-in French tickler just like the ads in comic books. But I'm sure this would be the sort of thing that one has no control over and it would happen during the most inappropriate circumstances: when you were being interviewed by the co-op board or when you were reciting the Four Questions at the seder, for example.

I don't have it bad. Yet. Dennis's friend has severe neuropathy. He is in such constant pain that he is taking morphine for it. My friend David had constant neuropathy. He couldn't button his shirts. He had to get special handles on the doors and for his mugs. Everything became a trial. With severe neuropathy, I don't suppose I'd be able to type anymore. I could always use a tape recorder and use my nose to push the buttons. I can't imagine how difficult putting on a condom could be, let alone masturbation. I wonder whether this is the sort of thing a visiting long-term home-care attendant would be conversant in.

According to AmFAR's *AIDS/HIV Treatment Directory*, "The first type, subacute and chronic demyelinating polyneuropathies, occurs relatively early in HIV infection, before susceptibility to major opportunistic infections, while the second type, predominantly sensory axonal polyneuropathy, develops as a late complication. The first is felt to have an autoimmune pathogenesis and, like subacute . . . or chronic idiopathic demyelinating polyneuropathy (CIPD), which develops in non-HIV-infected persons, responds favorably to plasma exchange and to glucocorticoids, with the former being the currently recommended treatment. The major morbidity of axonal predominantly sensory polyneuropathy relates to pain" (*AIDS/HIV Treatment Directory*, AmFAR, Vol. 6, No. 1, p. 73).

Translation: You're riding on bald tires. Your brake shoes are shot, and your shock absorbers have gone to hell. What you really need is a Midas muffler for myelin. After seeing *Lorenzo's Oil* I thought that maybe if Susan Sarandon were my mother, she would have come up with some nutritional supplement that could cure neuropathy, foil prejudice, halt nuclear proliferation, and lead to world peace. And then I realized the AIDS community already came up with its version of Lorenzo's Oil years ago: It's called AL721 and it didn't work.

Neuropathy hits the hands and feet first because they have the longest nerve cells. Remember all that stuff from high-school biology about neurons and axons and the myelin sheath? Who would expect to be using it twenty-odd years later?

I assume I have the mild form of neuropathy. I'm not in any major pain. Yet.

Everyone has advice for me. Chris says take vitamin B. Stan told me he thought it was part of the HIV thing, weird sensations in the feet and the hands. He didn't think it was necessarily caused by drugs. For all I know, it could be a consequence of lousy T-cells.

Last year I got the bogus ddC from the local buyers' club that they pulled off the market. The dosage was variable: I suppose they hadn't yet perfected the amount of baby laxative to use as filler. I figured it was bogus when I got neuropathy from the real thing. So now I'm trying peptide T from the local buyers' club to offset the side effects I should have gotten in the first place. Unfortunately for me, the local buyers' club has no money-back guarantee, no bulk discount, no cents-off coupons in the *PWA Newsline*. Although they don't take insurance or my Chubb LifeAmerica Prescription Drug Program, they do take Visa and American Express.

My doctor suggested I try peptide T for neuropathy. It's the coolest drug to take, with the neatest method of delivery. You squirt it up your nose: left nostril, right nostril, then left, not unlike nitrates of days of yore. This is a hell of a lot easier than spending twenty minutes with a leaky nebulizer, sucking up aerosol pentamidine. You're not supposed to hold your head back, because then it would drip down your throat. Instead, I hold my head upright and generally sneeze or have it drip down my nose.

Peptide T is also supposed to be good for mental alertness. I think it's failing universally because it has done absolutely nothing for my neuropathy and I keep forgetting to take it. I assume it would make a good dance-floor drug: Hang your inhaler on a chain around your neck and sniff it as the mirrored disco balls turn round and round and as Marky Mark fails to remove his shirt for the fiftieth time.

Having given up ddI and ddC, I'm stuck with AZT, which I've been taking for the past three years. It looks as if I've exhausted the current supply of FDA-approved drugs. My extremely good friend Jan, who gives the very best advice on absolutely everything and has incredibly bad judgment when it comes to his own relationships, has been in an observational database study for the past four years. Every six months he tells a tough gray-haired grandmother how many times he has jerked off in the past six months; how many times he's had cluster sex at a sex club or in the bushes at the Fenway in Boston; how many fingers he's inserted into anuses (others' and his own); how many partners he has had; how many steam-room erections he has produced and/or inspired; and so on. Surprisingly enough, quite a few of the subjects are still around after four years. One of the benefits of the study is a seminar on advances in AIDS care held by the physician leading the study. At the last seminar, the doctor stated that AZT was effective for from eighteen months to two years, and after that point it may serve only to increase the likelihood of getting lymphoma, which sort of terrifies me, especially after reading Paul Taylor's obituary in *The New York Times*. This was Paul Taylor the irritating art critic as opposed to

Paul Taylor the talented dancer and choreographer. Paul died of lymphoma. He was supposed to outlive me. I always assumed that he would dance on my grave, or, at the very least, write an irritating critical appraisal of my work. The last time I saw him was at Ron Vawter's performance piece about Roy Cohn and Jack Smith, which has received countless accolades, although for the life of me I can't understand why anyone would want to see a performance piece about Roy Cohn, the most evil homosexual in all history, although James Woods's performance on HBO did intrigue me and I probably would have seen it if I had premium cable, and I was exceptionally rude to Paul. The Jack Smith portion of the evening was important and historical and relentlessly dull to me, and I was appalled, even though it was my best friend John Weir's birthday and a large group of us had gone at his request, and when I saw Paul Taylor as the performance was letting out, he smiled and I just shrieked and left.

I knew he was positive. We were boyfriends for approximately three weeks several eons ago; I think it was sometime during the Jurassic era, shortly before the invention of fire and high-fidelity stereophonic sound. After encouraging me to accelerate the course of our relationship, Paul dumped me abruptly and completely, claiming we were "from different milieus," a locution that proved tautological; unregretfully, I have absolutely nothing in common with someone capable of using this locution without irony. Paul Taylor was infinitely inventive and infinitely cruel: He was the first person with call-waiting to put me on hold and then forget about me. But it was too late to reconcile my own personal difficulties with Paul Taylor and attain closure: Now he was dead from lymphoma.

Jan also found out at the seminar that patients generally get neuropathy after a year of ddC or ddI. I had probably taken in various doses and formulations bogus ddC, ddC Classic, and New ddI for about a year, so this seems to be par for the course. According to Rich Lynn of Treatment Action Group, reporting on the 1992 International AIDS Conference in Amsterdam, "I would swear that some of these investigators were happy when they discovered that their drug caused neuropathy. Neuropathy seems to be regarded as a surrogate marker for efficacy." Surrogate markers are not what fake law-school students use to highlight their stolen textbooks; they are alternative methods of judging a treatment's effectiveness. The only direct marker used in the earliest studies of AIDS drugs was the clinical endpoint, otherwise known as death.

After the first signs of neuropathy I immediately stopped ddC. I switched back to ddI, the less-desirable drug, because it had to be taken on an empty stomach and ground up into powder with a mortar and pestle that I sometimes neglected to carry with me in my backpack (I hear Hoffmann-La Roche is currently working on a new formulation that's smaller and fizzes like Alka-Seltzer), but the tingling remained. I waited a week, and then a month, for the ddC to wash out of my system. I tried a lower dose of ddI. No dice. My fingers and feet still gave off these tiny flashes as if I were being attacked by Disney-animated sprites. I tend to doubt that AZT is doing anything other than transforming my internal organs into some toxic-waste dump: I've clinically progressed in terms of dropping below 200 T-cells, although I've never looked better.

In the words of Huey Lewis, "I want a new drug."

Ideally, I want to take an antiretroviral and an immune modulator in one, sort of like Certs, the breath and candy mint.

The next nucleoside analogue that is currently in expanded access, d4T, can also cause peripheral neuropathy. Looks like a dead-end street to me.

FLT might be the next drug. I met Jeremy at the gym a few years ago before he switched to Better Bodies and then switched back to Chelsea Gym. He told me he was taking FLT, but he wouldn't return my phone calls because he was "emotionally unavailable" because he was in some twelve-step program: Does this make sense? I would like to find out how he's doing on FLT, since he obviously doesn't want to have sex with me, but it doesn't look too likely, since I haven't seen him at the gym for five months, which incidentally is not a good surrogate marker. I subsequently learned that he had died.

At this point I'm ready for anything: I'm ready for acupuncture. I'm ready for aromatherapy. I'm ready for meditation. I'm ready for arcane Eastern therapies. I'm ready for shark cartilage and bitter-melon enemas. I'm ready for deep-tissue massage. I'm even ready for therapy. I've always been ready for therapy; there just doesn't seem to be any time. I feel that I'm getting crazier and crazier. When I threw up in the middle of the new Woody Allen movie, I'm sure it was a combination of eating a natural cereal from Los Angeles that had enough undigestible natural fiber to create a ream of recycled paper and those extremely rough camera angles. *Husbands and Wives* was not unlike a ninety-minute ride on the Cyclone at Coney Island; I thought it was the beginning of the end.

I've had the beginning-of-the-end feeling at least once a week for the past seven years. I'll have a mild sore throat that doesn't go away and I'll think, "This is the beginning of the end." Or I will be a little congested and find that I don't have the full seventeen-gallon capacity in my lungs and I'll be convinced that I fucked up the last time I inhaled pentamidine and I have a PCP breakthrough. Or I'll get anxious and nervous and start to doubt my sanity and wonder if this is me or perhaps the first foreshadowings of dementia and I'll think, "This is the beginning of the end." Or I'll read an obituary in *The New York Times* of a playwright named Scott McPherson who died at thirty-three, younger than I am now and I'll think, "This is the beginning of the end." Or my hands will buzz and maybe I will get a brief stabbing pain in my feet and I'll think, "This is the beginning of the end."

Peptide T seems useless. My doctor recently suggested taking Elavil, an antidepressant, before I go to sleep. It may reduce neuropathy; the mechanism is unknown. I'm totally paranoid about antidepressants because my father was a manic–depressive who took lithium carbonate and my deranged friend Richard in San Francisco is on Elavil: For some bizarre reason, I associate the medication with mental illness, not a pleasant association at all. I think I've figured it out: You don't get rid of it, but you just don't care anymore. In which case, maybe a postprandial pitcher of vodka stingers would work just as well.

••

Oh, the vagaries of publishing! By the time QW published "Cocktails from Hell" (pp. 109–14) the piece was obsolete. The delightfully scatterbrained AIDS editor asked me for a contribution shortly before her vacation. I dashed off a first draft from my nefarious and multitudinous notes over a weekend and faxed it to her. Before she left for two weeks in Ireland, she told me vaguely that the piece was too digressive. I asked for specific advice on where to cut. When she returned, she had more pressing matters to take care of. A week later, I went to Montreal for a week's vacation. I returned to find that she had been dismissed. The files were a shambles. The new AIDS editor, a pleasant-enough fellow who was a little high-strung (he was rumored to hum "I don't like Mondays" as he butchered pieces and inserted the correct political slant), had lost the original. I dropped off another copy. By then QW was covering the International AIDS Conference in Amsterdam. The new AIDS editor recalled going over the piece once. When pressed, he also had some oblique criticisms. Unable to get anything specific, I told him I would cut it down to a thousand words. I figured the full-blown version with its full-blown AIDS anxiety would eventually appear in some Chapbook from Hell. He appeared pleased with the results. Then, of course, one day before deadline, seven weeks after I had originally submitted the piece, he called me with a thousand and one useless questions. He was treating it like a serious science piece, as opposed to a touchie-feelie-hysterical spasm of nerves. I had a typically deranged author hissy fit and QW finally ran the piece two months after I'd written it. And I was extremely pissed because by the time the piece eventually reached the light of day it was obsolete because I was off ddI and ddC because I had developed minor neuropathy.

"Needles and Pins" never made it into QW. By the time I finished it, QW itself was obsolete.

Ron Vawter died of AIDS-related causes on April 16, 1994.

Notes
on Sex

The worst thing about being a celebrity is that anonymous sex is no longer possible.

Gore Vidal once said never turn down an opportunity to have sex or be on television. Keep this in mind the next time Robin Byrd invites you to be on her cable show.

Always be aware of your physical placement in relationship to potential sex partners: on the checkout line at the Food Emporium, on the E train, and especially at a Queer Nation Kiss-In.

It is bad taste to make a date at a memorial, especially with the deceased's ex-lover.

Never have sex with your boss during your annual review, unless you are a prostitute and he is a pimp and this is a performance review.

Don't get annoyed when you find your two best friends had sex while you were on the telephone, unless, of course, you are only annoyed that they didn't invite you to join in.

In sex, quality is more important than quantity. And I'm not a size queen.

When someone tells you he doesn't like blowjobs, that's just a nice way of saying he's not interested. If this happens, one is advised to rise from a kneeling position.

If someone tells you he is attracted only to uncut dick, he is not necessarily anti-Semitic. He is, however, politically incorrect to the nth degree, and you can feel free to call him on it, loudly, in public, especially if he is sitting in the next pew at Congregation Beth Simchat Torah during the High Holy Days.

Sex is a good way to kill half an hour while your Lean Cuisine is in the oven. With the prevalence of microwaves, such so-called "fast food" sex has reached frenetic and exhausting proportions.

The more sex you have, the more you want.

Boring sex is better than no sex at all.

Sex can be used to reduce anxiety while waiting for election-night returns, to see if your co-op bid has been accepted, or to find out if you had a bad reaction to Septra.

Sex with a stranger is more exciting than sex with a known quantity.

It is considered rude to take a phone call in the midst of a sexual encounter, unless it's your agent, your crazy friend long distance from San Francisco who is threatening a suicide pact with you unbeknownst to you, or the pizza delivery man who can't get into your apartment because the downstairs door is locked. Your mother, however, should leave a message on the machine.

Don't forget to introduce the trick that you met at the leather bar to your roommate before you go off in his two-door convertible Chevy to a place you've never been before so your roommate can identify the trick in a lineup.

The wonderful thing about same-sex relationships is that it is possible to be attracted to both members of a couple simultaneously. There are n factorial possibilities and combinations of couplings and jealousy, all leading to disastrous results.

Don't invite someone over for a threesome without first checking with your partner to see if he is interested.

The advantage of going to his apartment for sex is that you can leave whenever you want. If he comes over to your place, he could be there indefinitely. Some people don't pick up on subtle hints: an obvious yawn, changing into pajamas, going to the corner bodega for a quart of milk, walking him to the subway. Also, if the guy from the phone-sex line turns out to be an axe murderer, he will be left with the problem of how to dispose of the body. If he comes to your apartment, he can simply leave it there.

The major disadvantage of going to his apartment for sex is that you have to dress. You don't always have cab fare. You may need to go to a cash machine, and not all of them are open at three in the morning. You may need to bring over your own poppers. You may need to carry your contact-lens case, Water Pik, dental floss, and mortar and pestle if you're on ddI. If it's raining, it can be hell getting a cab, even at three in the morning on Broadway and Fifty-second. He may be an early riser. He may have a dog. He may have a roommate. He may have a homicidal lover.

Try to agree on the behavior before you go with your boyfriend to a sex club such as Prism Gallery. You don't want to be screamed at when you suggest a threesome and he says he's not interested in having sex with you. Make sure you know the layout. It can be embarrassing having sex in a private cubicle and then finding out that he was watching you the entire time through the peephole without your knowledge. It can be distressing if he starts complaining that you never kiss him the way you kissed that stranger that night.

New York City is a land of bottoms. England is a land of bottoms. The entire universe is filled with bottoms. If you are a top, you will always be in demand. If you have a boyfriend, you should alternate playing top. It makes no sense to have those endless arguments about who was bottom for the past three nights in a row. Consider using a paperweight to mark the most recent position, or a reversible sweater. The situation can get mighty slippery, especially if lubrication has been applied.

Sex without ejaculation is like leaving a film noir ten minutes before the end.

There is no sex without guilt.

If it isn't in *The New Joy of Gay Sex*, then I'd rather not hear about it.

••

I was attempting a cross between Susan Sontag's "Notes on 'Camp'" and Fran Lebowitz's "Notes on Trick." I had been working on this piece for a few months when I was asked to review The New Joy of Gay Sex *for* QW. *I immediately agreed.* The New Joy of Gay Sex *was basically review-proof: It was bound to be a best-seller. I was sure Julia Roberts would star in the movie and it would gross more than $100 million. Yet oddly enough, I became totally terrified at the awesome responsibility I had accepted. To write a fair review, wouldn't I have to perform each and every act described in the pages? Why couldn't I have gotten an easier as-*

signment, like reviewing The Fannie Farmer Cookbook or The Encyclopaedia Britannica?

I was so overwhelmed that I found I was unable to read the book. Instead, I merely tacked on the final note to my ongoing "Notes on Sex" and submitted it as a review, just as QW began its indefinite hiatus.

Waiting for the End of the World

1. Writing as Procrastination

Thomas Alva Edison said that genius is 1 percent inspiration and 99 percent perspiration. As every writer knows, writing is 1 percent inspiration and 99 percent procrastination—unless, of course, you're the embarrassingly prolific Ethan Mordden, the gay Joyce Carol Oates, who has no doubt perfected the art of writing in his sleep and is probably polishing off an essay on Greta Garbo as he naps through another session, hopefully not this one. Or John Preston, who is editing his tenth anthology this year as we speak, *At Nine: Gay Men Talk about Their Fourth-Grade Teachers.*

This is how I write. I sit down at the table and power up the PC. I notice that the flowers in the vase are drooping. I go out to the Korean deli across the street and pick up a fresh bouquet. I carefully arrange them. I power up the PC. I notice that there is an inch of dust on the mantel in the next room. I spend an hour or so Pledge-ing the mantelpiece, the television, the VCR, the

Delivered as a talk at the Publishing Triangle Writers' Weekend, New York City, October 18, 1992; published in Art & Understanding, *January/February 1993.*

stereo, the CD player, the lamp. I write my mother a letter. I power up the PC. Getting into a comfortable position, I inadvertently kick a Combat bait tray, which reminds me to check the sticker on the refrigerator, which tells me that I haven't changed my roach repellent in seven months. I go out to the drugstore on Eighth Avenue and get some fresh Combat. I turn off the PC because it's lunchtime. I call the phone-sex line and listen to the messages, stopping only after I've gone back to the message I had left eight hours earlier. With a start, I realize that I've forgotten to pay the rent and it's already the fifth. I frantically search for my checkbook. Half an hour later, I find it in the vegetable crisper. I write the check. I mail it at the post office. On the way, I pick up my mail, which includes the latest issues of *Vanity Fair* and *Advocate Men*. Two hours later, I power up the PC. I go to the cabinet for a teacup. The shelf paper needs to be replaced. I reline the shelves. I write my mother another letter. I turn on the PC. My fingers are tense. Worried about carpal tunnel syndrome, I go to the gym to stretch out and relax. I come home and write a letter to my ex-boyfriend. I masturbate. I read a promotional brochure from World Gym on the Upper West Side and decide to join immediately (the special ends in five hours) because it is open twenty-four hours a day, so if I ever feel the urge to write at three-thirty in the morning I will always have an alternative. I realize I'm almost out of paper and take a train downtown to my favorite stationery store and buy a ream of paper and a magazine to read on the subway back home. I turn on my PC. I remember that I haven't done my pentamidine in three weeks. I take the machine down from the shelf and power it up. I can't find the syringes in the bathroom. I clean the tub. I masturbate. I write my mother another letter. I throw out all three letters to my mother because at this point in my life I'm not particularly fond of her.

I'm still hazy as to how I was able to write two books. I think a dog named Sam may have dictated them to me while I slept.

2. Wasting Time

On the other hand, there's this little voice in the back of my head (I've named it "Mom") that's constantly telling me not to waste time. We're living in AIDS time. We're living in dog years. I may look a little like Drew Barrymore in *Poison Ivy*, but physically I'm a lot closer to Meryl Streep in the final reel of *Death Becomes Her*. The clock is ticking, constantly ticking, like one of those annoying Swatches that you bury in the next room under the socks in the laundry bag when you bring home a trick but you can still hear it ticking, ticking, ticking: It's like having sex to a metronome. Life is a commercialless episode of "Sixty Minutes" complete with stopwatch, and I don't want to be tied up in tubes, unable to avoid Andy Rooney's homespun homilies on my deathbed as Shana Alexander dukes it out with the devil for possession of my immoral soul.

In a sense everything I do, save work on my stillborn novel and moribund play, is a waste of time: waiting for that epiphany in the Chelsea Gym steam room, writing a review of the *Chore of Gay Sex* for *QW*, shuffling papers at work, writing this piece. I take minor solace that it may eventually end up in my posthumous collection of random pieces, *Life in Hell*. I wonder if they have fax machines in hell so I can get editorial advice for the final page proofs; this probably won't be necessary, as from past experience I'm sure hell will be filled with editors.

3. Hard Questions

The clock is ticking and there are hard questions that require immediate answers.

Should I buy the co-op in Chelsea and risk getting booted to Bailey House when I lose my job?

Should I go on disability when my T-cells drop below 50?

Should I learn Braille now or later?

•   •   •

It looks as if I can safely retire Proust to the bookshelves, along with nixing reading *The Divine Comedy* in the original Italian. Do I really have to see a once-in-a-lifetime twenty-hours-with-no-intermission theatrical experience presented at the Brooklyn Academy of Music in an armory, sitting on a bench of nails, with my bare feet placed gingerly on a sea of broken glass? It's only $160, unreserved. In a word, no. With a declining T-cell count and concurrently shrinking lifespan, it's not inconceivable that Neil Simon's next might be a once-in-a-lifetime experience for me.

I still have to fight this Pavlovian response to be outside whenever it's sunny, because I grew up in Syracuse, New York, the cloudiest city in the continental U.S. save Seattle. Writers relish bad weather. I was particularly happy we had so many rainy days this summer. This has nothing at all to do with the fact that I didn't purchase a share on Fire Island this summer.

My revised goal in life remains to write five books, preferably published during my lifetime, and reach forty. I'm banking on the hope that I just may be too bitter to die.

4. Helpful Hints

I have a few helpful hints for aspiring writers with potentially terminal illnesses.

Carry a pad and pencil everywhere. The best ideas occur when you're stuck in the tunnel on the E train en route to Queens, trapped on the Stair Master for twenty-four minutes, or pinned against the wall of a back room in the East Village, waiting patiently for someone who looked extremely attractive half an hour and three beers ago and probably will never come.

Laptops are useful in dark environments such as the Prism Gallery: Make sure you have one with a backlit screen.

And finally, buy on credit.

5. Role Models

There are role models to follow. My favorite example of the hysterical output of a condemned man is Anthony Burgess, who, when falsely diagnosed with brain cancer, wrote five books in a single year in an attempt to support his soon-to-be widow. Andy Warhol dictated an exceedingly bad novel into a tape recorder over the course of twenty-four hours. Isaac Asimov, who used to pause at regular intervals to slap together a literary greatest-hits collection (*Opus 100*, *Opus 200*, etc.), once wrote a story while sitting in the display window of a bookstore. If only I had their stamina! It took me practically four months to write a will, and it's not as if I own anything. I'm sure I'll never commit suicide, because it would take me too long to write the proper note.

6. Anxiety as Fuel

No matter what I do or think, AIDS remains the subtext, the subliminal humming of that perpetual-motion machine with six rechargeable Energizer batteries hidden in the base. AIDS is always in the background, constant as the beating of my heart. If the virus itself hasn't yet passed the blood-brain barrier, the idea of the virus has already poisoned my mind. I vacillate between periods of mild anxiety and total hysteria. It takes a while getting used to being HIV-positive. I think it took me two years to modulate my response to a somewhat manageable level of abject terror. I was lucky to have had the time to adjust. Far too many people haven't.

Anxiety is my fuel, my motivation. Ideally, I would have liked to have gotten a false-positive test result when I was ten. Imagine how productive I would have been with this constant high level of anxiety, uncontrollable by any known psychopharmaceutical.

7. The Paradox of the Condemned Man

Back in high school when I was a math nerd, I was fascinated by the paradox of the condemned man. A prisoner was told that he would be executed at some time in the next ten days but on a day that he wouldn't expect it. He reasoned that they couldn't kill him on the tenth day, because he would expect it. They couldn't kill him on the ninth day, because he knew they couldn't kill him on the tenth day and therefore would expect to be killed on the ninth. Reasoning backward, he was able to deduce that he couldn't be killed at all on any of the days. Thus, of course, when he was executed on the seventh day, he didn't expect it.

My death sentence was announced years ago. I sit here condemned by a mutating virus and a government that refuses to allocate adequate resources toward finding a cure. But everyone is condemned to death the moment they are born. The only certainty is the uncertainty of the date they will expire.

HIV-positive people can be stable for years. I was probably infected ten years ago. I've been HIV-positive for more than a quarter of my life. So far, aside from a few minor dermatological problems, I've suffered only side effects.

There's a part of me that knows that I'll never die. There's a part of me that knows better.

8. Good Vegetable/Bad Vegetable

Toward the end of *Catch-22*, Yossarian has a telling conversation with Major Danby:

> "I think I'd like to live like a vegetable and make no important decision."
> "What kind of vegetable, Danby?"
> "A cucumber or a carrot."
> "What kind of cucumber? A good one or a bad one?"
> "Oh, a good one, of course."

"They'd cut you off in your prime and slice you up for a salad."

Major Danby's face fell. "A poor one, then."

"They'd let you rot and use you for fertilizer to help the good ones grow."

"I guess I don't want to live like a vegetable, then," said Major Danby with a smile of sad resignation.

Here are my options: Do I want to die a slow, protracted death, ending up on life support in some sterile hospital, half-man, half-machine? Or do I want to die instantly, an absurd death, run over by a laundry truck, suffocated in my own vomit, overdosed on morphine, taunted by Gary Indiana lisping bad reviews of my books?

Quite honestly, neither.

Do I want to be buried six feet underground in a coffin and slowly decompose and end up as food for worms? Or do I want to be cremated, consumed by fire in a preview of hell, have my flesh destroyed beyond recognition and end up in an urn on someone's mantelpiece or tossed into a body of water and eventually fertilize the floor of the ocean?

Let's face it, both alternatives suck.

The final wishes of an atheist are ultimately meaningless. I mean, I *would* like to be cremated after any salvageable organs have been donated to right-wing Republicans and religious fundamentalists (because I'm really not bitter after all).

But ultimately it isn't my concern.

9. Vegetables

I definitely don't want to end up a vegetable.

Perhaps my greatest fear is the loss of lucidity. Initially, writing is an extremely private act. Not even boyfriends are allowed to look over your shoulder when you're typing that first draft. Unconditional approval is necessary at the early stages of the work. I'd rather not have anyone read what I've written until the paperback has been reissued twenty years after initial publication: Criticism can cast a pall on one. In any event, for the first several drafts, the work must undergo the subjectivity of self-examination. No one else can really help: not the writing group from Bennington, not the dyslexic therapist, not the former best friend from high school who now lives in Portland, and not the writer's mother. Reading your own work can often be surprising: Work that seems excellent on one day may seem execrable on another. Humor is particularly subjective.

But when I lose the ability to examine my own work critically, it will be time to stop writing altogether. You ultimately can't depend on anyone but yourself to review your writing.

10. Conclusion

So on the one hand I'll continue to procrastinate, pretending that I don't have a potentially life-threatening illness. This is known as denial. On the other hand, I'll write as fast as I can, as if I had only one year to live. Anxiety is the best fuel for me. Everyone should write out of desperation: as if there is only one year to live, except, of course, for the high priestesses of style like Edmund White, who should take as long as necessary to perfect their sentences. I don't think I'm likely to write a TV sit-com pilot on spec in the near future. But then again, if I ever get that elusive Chelsea co-op, I may end up writing copy on the back of Post Toasties.

My silly data-processing job provides health care and enough money so I don't have to worry about the fact that *QW* pays four weeks after publication, and I can basically write whatever I want, contingent upon the fact that it may or may not get printed. I feel a constant low-level guilt that I should quit my job and work full-time to end the AIDS crisis and volunteer for AIDS organizations in all my spare time and stop that narcissistic gym-going and pathological flirting and burn out and do research for ACT UP's Treatment and Data Committee, and even writing is a waste of time, because writing doesn't have the power to save a single life. I should be out there on the front lines like Larry Kramer founding activist organizations and denouncing them in due time.

In *Screening History*, Gore Vidal mentions that there is no such thing as a "famous novelist" because "Adjective is inappropriate to noun. How can a novelist be famous, no matter how well known he may be personally to the press, when the novel itself is of no consequence to the civilized, much less to the generality?" Why persist in writing, a hopelessly bourgeois act, an act of vanity?

I write because it's the most difficult thing that I know how to do. I write because I feel I have something important to say. I write because it's arguably the only thing I can do well.

••

I wrote this for a gay and lesbian writers' conference organized by the Publishing Triangle and CUNY's Center for Lesbian and Gay Studies. The topic was "AIDS Time." This panel was slapped together when the organizers realized they had forgotten to include an AIDS panel. I spent a few weeks refining this piece. I want to thank Joe Keenan for inspiring the title of John Preston's anthology. I felt hopelessly pseudointellectual by citing Joseph Heller, as if I were pretending to write a piece seriously grounded in the literature. Why not Sontag? Why not James? Why not Proust? Luckily I had just stumbled onto Gore Vidal's latest essays. I was extremely annoyed when I discovered that I was the only one on the panel who had prepared specifically for this session. James Turcotte, who had reminded me that I had read too long at George Stambolian's memorial reading, read from his diaries. The other panelists spoke off the top of their heads. One of the editors of Art & Understanding *was on the panel. He asked if I would submit my essay. It was run in the January/February 1993 issue, and later reprinted for the Berlin Conference issue.*

I learned tht James Turcotte had died when the Publishing Triangle reprinted his address posthumously. John Preston died of AIDS-related complications on April 28, 1994.

Warts
from
Hell

I have approximately six hundred and forty-seven warts on my left hand, and four hundred and seventy-two warts on my right. This has absolutely nothing to do with my masturbatory practices. My extremely good friend Jan, who is better than Dear Abby, Ann Landers, and Susie Sexpert rolled into one, would say that I've been kissing a lot of frogs trying to find my own Jewish-American Prince, and maybe given one or two handjobs too many in the process. This is not the case. HIV is not the only virus I harbor. To be truthful, the actual number of warts on my hands is closer to forty-nine, which nonetheless is still enough to make strong men grow pale.

I've been plagued by warts on my hands since I moved to New York in 1979. I assume this predates my HIV, but I could be wrong. I used to wait until four or five of them had reached a certain, shall we say, size, and then have a delightful visit with my dermatologist, an epicene rice queen who kept photos of his estranged wife and three daughters on his desk. Dr. Q lived in a large one-family unit in Nassau County that he shared with an ever-changing set of Oriental college-student boarders. He had a sense of humor drier than his own parched skin; he would burst into drunken tears at Uncle Charlie's and show pocket-size copies of the photos on his desk at work to any stranger who would look. After a wry comment, he would anesthetize the area of my hand and then burn the warts out with an instrument that I expect Laurence Olivier used to rehearse his Nazi film roles. This in turn stimulated several all-but-invisible wartlets on my hands, which soon grew to take the place of those eradicated. For years the number of warts on my hands remained a scientific constant, akin to the speed of light or the sum-total mass of a closed system. Now it's out of control.

More recently, Dr. Q preferred to dip a Q-tip into a Styrofoam cup he had filled with liquid nitrogen and then press the Q-tip on the wart. Oddly enough, this produced a burning sensation. Later a blister would appear. When this healed, unfortunately, the wart generally remained. Some say my warts will end in fire, some say my warts will end in ice.

In my present state, I am so wart-besotted that I fear I would do damage if I inserted any single digit up any ass, even my own: At this point I don't have a single wart-free finger. I am loath to shake a stranger's hand, except of course a business associate, for fear of contagion. Have my hands become the literal embodiment of my generalized fear of HIV infection?

Surprisingly, they are less of a pain than an annoyance. They generally don't interfere with touch-typing or gym workouts— although for a while I had two warts on the side of my fourth finger, two large ones, and this caused moderate pain when I was holding hands with various strangers in my capacity as a marshal, blocking nonexistent traffic during David Wojnarowicz's memorial procession through the East Village. Those warts magically disappeared, perhaps giving some credence to the concept that they could be willed away, although the rest have remained, and redoubled.

I hold the mottled portrait of Dorian Gray in my hands.

When I would visit Jan, the first thing he'd ask is, "How are your hands?"

"Fine," I'd reply.

"Let me see them," he'd demand. I'd offer Jan my hands, placing them palms up in his. He would inspect them with mock seriousness. "A little better," he would attest.

"Actually, I think they're a little worse."

"As long as they're not interfering with your workouts."

"Sure. I pretend I get them from pull-ups." They are occasionally mistaken for calluses.

I suppose I'm just as vain as the next male homosexual who goes to a gymnasium one short block away from Barneys, a store so intimidating that I have yet to actually enter this haberdashery for fear of inadvertently buying a $1,075 Versace knit shirt marked down to $850. Don't ask me why, but *this* is the piece I didn't want to be published during my lifetime. For some reason, I've always viewed my warts as the outward physical manifestation of some deadly character flaw I should have long ago eradicated through a concentrated act of self-control. My warts shame me. I hold my hands tightly balled up, as if to deny their presence. I willfully ignore them, as if by ignoring them they would cease to exist. It took me two weeks to tell my boyfriend about them (although he already knew). I told him I was HIV-positive fifteen minutes after we met.

Is it because the warts are the most visible symptom of my declining immune system? Is it because I fear they may be wildly contagious (although it seems their contagion is confined to myself)? Or is it because they are *not particularly appealing* and might constitute a sexual *turn-off*?

I communicate sexually primarily by touching and kissing. With warts, my hands are rendered useless, two contaminated vessels with all the appeal of a rotting octopus. And before I adopted nightly cleanings with the Water Pik and Peridex, my gums from hell seemed to bleed spontaneously at the mere thought of arousal: How was I to kiss without dread? What was I left with: a buttoned-lipped peck on the cheek and a rubber-gloved full-body massage? Now that I've almost completely removed the possibility of human contact, am I left to fend for myself alone fully encased in plastic?

Perhaps my hands are only contagious to someone else with an even lower immune system. What am I to do? Ask for a T-cell count (are there home methods like home pregnancy tests?) before continuing without the same latex gloves that the cops wear when they're planning on arresting us?

There were long periods when I would visit my doctor every other week to get treated for my anal warts. My former physician, who purchased his condo with my insurance payments (my warts were listed as lien-holders on the deed), was totally bereft of a bedside manner. He died abruptly of AIDS, no doubt leaving his unknowing patients with an acute sensation of dislocation. My last two dentists are dead. In the nineties, divulging HIV status takes on a new perspective: The urban gay male worries less about transmission from his physician than whether or not he will survive him.

My doctor offered me various methods of treatments for the warts on my hands. One was salicyclic-acid plasters. Every night I was told to soak my hands in hot water, dry them, and then cut up pieces of the acid plaster to stick on top of my warts overnight. I could never find the tiny-spot Band-Aids at Duane Reade to cover them. If it's something I have to be vigilant at, chances are that I won't follow through. I'm just no good at anything more complicated than popping poisonous pills three or four times a day. I'm sure that injections, should they eventually become necessary, will be a major problem.

In December 1990 someone gave a presentation on human papilloma virus at an ACT UP meeting. HPV causes venereal warts; it is also linked to cervical cancer. The presenter suggested it was a good idea to get rid of anal and genital warts because of the risk of cancer. I had assumed that I still had some, because my warts always returned. Clearing up my anal warts seemed an exercise in futility, adding a few stitches to a Jacquard-knit shirt that was unraveled every night. My anus was in a semipermanent state of sexual retirement at the time. But learning of the threat of cancer, I decided I might as well invest in a brief bout of spring cleaning.

My doctor found one small wart and treated it with acetic acid. He also discovered that I had a singular hemorrhoid: I always thought they came in pairs, like M&Ms. He referred me to a well-known laser surgeon who I assumed restricted his practice to the nether regions for the warts on my hands. For fear of libel, I shall refer to him as Doktor Gluteus Maximus.

I visited Dr. G. M. during the Gulf war. Families and couples huddled in pain in the waiting room from post-op trauma or preexamination anxiety, as the missiles rained down on CNN. Dr. G. M. had cable. The waiting room was our own private Baghdad filled with war casualties of another sort.

I was in to see Dr. G. M. for my hands.

"Oh, and by the way, I had a few anal warts. My doctor treated one this week. You might as well check to make sure they are all gone." These famous last words will go down in my personal history like Napoleon's pep talk at Waterloo.

Dr. G. M. advertised "No bleeding. No pain." No way!

Remember the bleeding toilet in Francis Ford Coppola's *The Conversation*? That was my existence for the next ten days. I became intimate with all varieties of feminine-hygiene products; I was especially partial to Light Days panty liners. I developed a new appreciation for Tucks pads. My steps were measured and tiny, the steps of an octogenarian who recently had a hip replaced, as I walked the one-block distance to the nearest drugstore for additional supplies, hoping that I would make it back before incontinence struck again. Even farts were painful.

I took three sitz baths daily, hot water with Epsom salts. I eventually ended up using an entire year's worth of sick days in a matter of two weeks. Shouldn't I be saving some days for a bout of PCP?

Gluteus Maximus, M.D., charged outrageous amounts. His practice was nothing more than a medical mill. There was something bizarre about taking an EKG before local anesthesia. My insurance statements would code every item with a special code, which on the obverse side indicated that the amount billed exceeded the customary amount.

After my insurance paid the first bill, I found that Dr. Posterior administered a much higher grade of anesthesia.

The pharmacist asked me pointed questions after I presented him with my initial prescription for Darvon. "Are these for you? Why do you feel you need painkillers?"

Pained, I told him, bordering on hysteria, "I've just had some extremely painful surgery."

He immediately clammed up and filled the script. I saved one extra prescription he had written for Demerol, should I ever decide to finish *Final Exit*. Now it's useless: Prescriptions for controlled substances are good for only six months in the state of New York. I should have had it filled immediately. I could have sold them at the next Saint-at-Large party.

On my next visit to the Fanny Physician, he zapped the warts on my hands. It was another nightmare. I understood why they couldn't do this at the same time as my anal warts: I wouldn't be able to turn on the bathwater with my hands in swatches of bloody gauze. I decided to document my stigmata. I set the self-timer and took photos of myself with hands spread à la Jesus. This could have been that year's Christmas card, but I shuddered to think what I would say in the annual letter. It was more appropriate for Easter, anyway. I sent one copy of the photos to my friend in L.A. He did not respond for several years—or perhaps not responding served as his response?

On my third visit to the Butt Doctor one of his associates posed that lethal $64,000 question: "Have we checked your penis yet?"

Two hours later I hobbled home, my mummified penis swathed in layers of cotton. A testament to my monumental insensitivity, this particular laser treatment was relatively painless, save the concept. That night I joined my best friend in the entire world, John Palmer Weir, Jr., and his glamorous editor for a cele-bratory dinner at some swank establishment. My bathroom visits were as infrequent as humanly possible. For the next five days I had to unravel my new synthetic foreskin, bathe my penis daily in a solution of hydrogen peroxide, and then smear it with triple an-tibiotic solution before reswathing in cotton. This is one place I won't risk infection.

Compounding my problems, a desperate sexual contact around this time results in crabs. Don't ask me how. I somehow manage to coordinate the application of a pediculicide with my efforts at phallic hygiene. Although in the manner of the Jewish-American Princess which I aspire to be, I generally drop off my laundry, Jan, convinced that service laundry is done at lower temperatures to save money, insisted that I wash my sheets, towels, and underwear myself. The height of ludicrousness occurred one Sunday afternoon when I was hobbling to the Laundromat, cheeks clenched, and rushing back between cycles to bake an apple cake I had previously promised to celebrate John Weir's unscheduled appearance on the "CBS Evening News" with Dan Rather.

Six weeks after my first encounter with the Heinie Horror, it's time to check my ass again. The anal warts have already returned. I postpone surgery until the following Monday, because I have friends in from out of town over the weekend. The physician ex-presses amazement at how fast the warts have spread, even since my last visit. After surgery, I am out of work for another seven days, not including the weekend. At this point my reconstructed asshole is worth approximately $20,000. I decide to retire it. Like a brand-new Mercedes before its first scratch, I am reluctant to expose it to the possibility of any further abuse. Absolutely noth-ing goes up there, not even unscented toilet paper.

I decide to forgo future treatment. It's not worth it to me if I have to return every six weeks for another two weeks of unendur-able pain. I keep this in mind should chemotherapy be indicated in the future. My down-time was spectacularly unproductive: I couldn't read, I couldn't write, although in my Darvon-induced haze I decided to write my next novel based on the Pet Shop Boys' latest CD.

A few weeks later the Posterior Physician is indicted on several charges of medical fraud and abuse. It develops that he had been barred from practicing in several neighboring states. Unnecessary surgery is one of many accusations. Scurrilous pieces appear in the daily tabloids, accusing him of sexually abusing his employees. The Butt Van is impounded. But of course he's still in business, to this day, I assume.

This past year nothing seemed to work. Years ago I used a gelatinlike petroleum-based product called Efudex on my anal warts, applying it myself with a finger cot. Now my doctor suggests using Efudex on my hands, every night, after wearing down the warts with a pumice stone. I soak my hands in warm water for five minutes and then whittle them down with the stone until I bleed, which may be why I tend to do this only once a month. But I am a bit leery of Efudex. If I apply vanishing cream on my face every night, will I eventually disappear? If I put some Efudex on my hands and then so much as accidentally touch my penis, will my member be erased? My endless nightly ritual has once again been extended indefinitely: swallow and or snort nocturnal drug doses with the appropriate beverage, brush teeth, floss, Water Pik, soak hands, rub with pumice stone, apply Efudex to the places that aren't still bleeding, and then sleep, making sure that any masturbatory practices have already been completed.

My doctor also gives me a small razor. I can cut them off myself. It's only dead skin. But it's my own skin. I have already overcome the natural fear of sticking my fingers into my eyes: I wear contact lenses. With practice and necessity, I could probably learn how to inject drugs with a needle. But I can't bring myself to cut myself, except inadvertently, when I'm shaving. Scratch that method of suicide.

Leaving an ACT UP meeting one Monday night, I shake hands with my old friend Philip, the filmmaker/masseur/near clinically depressive whom I haven't seen in several months. "Eek!" he shrieks, dropping my hand as if it contains a lethal dose of radio-activity. "Those are warts! They're highly contagious!" If so, my boyfriend's body would be completely covered by them by now.

My friend Tom tells me that all I have to do is soak my hands in warm salt water, pat them dry, then cover my warts with garlic oil, put on a pair of large latex gloves, and sleep in them. How can I do this with a steady boyfriend? Won't the odor alone drive him away?

My doctor tells me I can always will them away.

I wonder whether sacrificing a chicken would help.

At an ACT UP meeting, I find out that some men in a hyper-icin trial have discovered that their anal warts have disappeared. I am, of course, ineligible for entry to this trial: something to do with some drug I almost took last February or another drug I attempted to take in August.

I decide to try laser therapy again, but only for my hands. The receptionist at my former dermatologist, who is currently in South America working on his septum, refers me to another dermatologist whom I'd gone to once five years ago when I had impetigo; his receptionist refers me to a dermatologist at N.Y.U. Medical Center who does laser surgery. This time I'm prepared. I take the day off from work. I buy vast quantities of groceries: I remember how it felt when the plastic grocery bags dug into my wound-mottled palms. I have my last gym workout. I go to the video store and rent all three Indiana Jones movies, all three Star Wars, and the entire Buckshot collection. Masturbating will be a chore. The night before, I visit the Prism Gallery and spend several hours not getting laid.

I trudge over to the hospital for my 8:30 A.M. appointment. The doctor's office is located on the extreme East Side, far past any subway lines. Downstairs in the lobby are newsstands with my favorite daily tabloids, screaming headlines about Amy Fisher and Joey Buttafuocco. I find the correct floor and wait. The receptionist hands me the form I am so accustomed to filling out. I indicate I am HIV-positive in the appropriate section, and list the drugs I am currently taking.

"What's Trental for?" asks the intern.

"It's an experimental treatment which supposedly reduces tumor necrosis factor in the bloodstream," I rattle off.

"Oh."

The intern looks at my hands. She is taken aback. There are many more warts than she had expected. "You know there's a very low chance of curing warts in someone who's HIV-positive?"

I know.

"Do you have AIDS yet, or are you—?"

"I'm asymptomatic as yet. Just lousy T-cells."

I forgot to take the before photo for my personal pathogenesis scrapbook. I forgot to count them. Is this denial?

The doctor comes in. He looks at my hands.

"There is a zero cure rate for HIV-positive people," he tells me.

"I suspected. I thought maybe once a year I could come," I say to myself.

"I can't in good conscience use laser surgery on these warts. I would leave you with hundreds of open wounds. You have a low immune system, and putting you at such an increased risk of infection would be unconscionable. Have you tried anything topical?"

"Nothing seems to work."

"I'm sorry, but there's nothing I can do. Oh, but you should avoid picking at them, it only makes them spread."

Thanks a lot.

I resolve to grind them down nightly with my pumice stone, a resolution I break that very night. Instead of laser surgery, I do the obvious alternative: I go shopping. I spend all the money I will receive in my imaginary AIDS-discrimination suit against the hospital, the intern, and the resident physician. I buy a leather jacket at Macy's and two pair of Calvin Klein undershirts, one of which was too small to wear but it was on sale—so how could I resist?—and two pair of pants at the Gap, duplicates of pairs I had purchased previously, so now I have one identical pair (I had to throw the other original out when I got too much fake blood on it when I was demonstrating in D.C. chained to the White House fence), and a nonstick rolling pin from Lechter's and a sifter, which my boyfriend promptly broke, and a large bottle of Duane Reade mouthwash, which is half the price of Scope, and some other stuff. I return home and play my messages from well-wishers who have called to comfort me after my surgery. The painkillers are neatly arrayed on the kitchen table. I return them to the bathroom cabinet and weep.

Remember how it felt when you were a kid gluing together a plastic model? When you were finished, you had some dried rubber cement stuck on your fingertips. Or you would pick your nose and end up with day-old mucus under your nails. Sometimes it would be stubborn, but eventually you could wash it off. Well, whenever I rub my fingers together, I feel the same type of physical deformations. Except it doesn't rub off. Ever.

The Day
From Hell

It starts off like any other day, but by the time it's over, you realize it has been the Day from Hell.

Part 1

The alarm rings at 6:45 A.M. Fuck the gym. I turn over and go back to sleep. I have carnal knowledge of my boyfriend at 8:15 A.M. I arrive at work at 9:30 A.M. I read the paper. Work is hell. We have an endless meeting about our hardware migration at 11:30 A.M. I talk to my best friend in the world, John P. Weir, for about an hour to recover from the meeting. I spend ninety minutes typing up memos and letters to vendors at 3:00 P.M. My best friend in the world, John P. Weir, calls me at 4:45 P.M. I meet the extremely loquacious Gil, everybody's favorite Chelsea real-estate agent, at 5:30 P.M. to look at apartments. The first is huge. Perfect for sex parties, remarks Gil. The second has a sauna. The third has a sunken living room with an iron railing. This is where you would put the handcuffs, Gil comments. Leaving the last apartment, we run into Bruce, whom I tricked with in 1981. He played the piano and talked too much. He offered to fuck me. I demurred. Not on the first date. He said there wasn't going to be a second date. His lover, Dale, is in the hospital. Dale isn't doing well. I assume Dale is the Dale who was the last person to fuck me without a condom, back in 1983. He slipped it in surreptitiously, and I complained, and later he said I had nothing to worry about because he was only a top. Later I find out it is a different Dale. At 7:30 P.M. I buy flowers to celebrate six months of hopeless misunderstanding and dysfunction with my boyfriend. At 7:45 P.M. sexual congress of a somewhat ambivalent nature takes place. I don't particularly feel like it after hearing about Dale. At 8:30 P.M. Binky asks, "What was that all about?" I explode in anger. At 9:15 P.M. he disappears for a "walk." I write letters and postcards. I talk to my friend Wayne at 10:30 P.M. I take a Xanax and go to sleep at 11:00 P.M. Binky returns at 11:30 P.M. and sleeps on the floor.

Part 2

I see my doctor at 1:30 P.M. He takes blood for T-cells and tests for toxoplasmosis, cytomegalovirus, and cryptosporidium.

He burns nine mollusca from my neck. I shouldn't touch them. They will blister, then scab.

He gives me a pneumonia shot in the arm, and a pentamidine shot in the ass. In the new office they will offer IV pentamidine in an infusion room that will have TVs. I'm not looking forward to that.

He gives me a shot of B_{12} in the arm.

I find out my last T-4 count was 105.

He recommends I try peptide T, a nasal spray, twice a day, from the PWA Health Group. He also recommends seeing an eye doctor once a year; twice a year when my count goes below 50. He gives me to referrals.

I go back to work.

After work, like an idiot, I go to the gym. My arm hurts.

Then I go to ACT UP for two hours. The phone tree is acti-
vated again.

I go to sleep. My arm hurts.

I hear a mouse fidgeting in the trash.

I get up at 3:00 A.M. and see the mouse in the trash.

I go to the A&P on Ninth Avenue and Fifty-fifth, which is
open twenty-four hours except for those rare occasions when you
actually need it at 3:00 in the morning. It is closed. I find some
poison at a Korean deli and throw it in the trash.

I wake up at 8:00 A.M. The mouse is dead or asleep in the trash.
Did the mouse eat the rest of the poison? Did it commit suicide?
It didn't leave a note. I double-bag the trash and throw it out.

After work I buy some glue traps, mouse poison, and bug
bombs.

Luis is in a morphine-induced coma. I met Luis three years ago
in ACT UP at a series of demos we had in Atlanta. He is dying of
lymphoma.

That night, I take a nap after dinner. I wake up at 11:00 P.M.
and go back to sleep at 11:30.

Part 3

I am down to 90 T-cells. I call to enroll in a vaccine trial. I am
placed on a waiting list. They never reach my name. I don't panic.
I've been this low before and I've bounced back. I feel I won't
bounce back. Last time I had a cold. I was retested the following
week. I reached for my checkbook and the doctor worriedly said,
"There will be no charge for this," which made me even more
nervous.

Part ...

It starts out like any other day, but by the time it's over, you realize

The
Canals
of Mars

Next time I'll remember my sunglasses.

I've always hated sunglasses. I admit mirrored motorcycle shades can be sexy, but only because I imagine the brightest, clearest blue eyes behind them. Generally, the wearer of said eye apparel, perhaps confusing a statuesque physique with a statuesque demeanor, will remain immobile long enough to function as an aid to personal hygiene and grooming. I have on several occasions, upon failing to elicit any human response, used an impassive person's glasses to determine whether a piece of celery or a pubic hair was stuck in my teeth, all the time loudly commenting on my dilemma.

Sunglasses function primarily as a barrier, a way of avoiding someone's glance. I never know whether the wearer of sunglasses is looking at me, through me, or beyond me, at the skinny blond in the red kerchief barreling through the crowd on roller blades. Sunglasses are just one more layer of hypocrisy to me. I still recall with some nausea the ridiculous fashion a few years back of wearing frames with regular glass to appear intellectual, and knowing someone who would wear contacts beneath such glasses. I suppose there may be some protective value to sunglasses, but frankly, I prefer crow's-feet to raccoon eyes.

Only now my eyes are saucers. My pupils could swallow you. It's a look: sexy, but incompetent. Margaret Keane herself could have painted me as another sad-eyed orphan as I stagger home from my ophthalmologist, located on swank Park Avenue, an impressive but not particularly convenient address. It's a gorgeous day. I'd feel guilty if I took a cab in such clement weather, if I could find one without running into it. The sun is shining brightly and even the cars look freshly bleached: television ads for Tide or household cleanser. The sun is deadly and I feel like a vampire as I try to leap from one building shadow to the next. If only Dr. F. took evening appointments, preferably when the moon wasn't full.

I am here to see Dr. Judith F. on the advice of my physician. Given my current health status, it would behoove me to visit an eye doctor specializing in HIV twice a year. I have to watch out for cytomegalovirus retinitis. About 95 percent of the population has been exposed to CMV. It can lead to blindness in people with impaired immune systems. The generally accepted treatment involves implanting a Hickman catheter in the chest and daily or thrice-weekly infusions of an antiviral. This treatment only stabilizes the condition; any vision loss is permanent. There is an experimental treatment called intravitreal implants, where smaller doses of the drug are delivered directly to the eye. A single implant can last several months. Implants avoid the common risk of infection at the catheter sight.

I haven't had regular eye checkups in years. The last time I saw an optometrist three years ago I ended up paying one month's rent for a pair of designer frames that still cause comment.

In Dr. F's waiting room are elderly ladies and frail young men with earrings.

Her office wall is covered with medical degrees from N.Y.U., which somehow makes me feel smug. I had taped my N.Y.U. degree to the bathroom door. The edges curled after a succession of showers. I think I lost it in my last move.

The doctor is wearing a purple pantsuit. Photos of her son and daughter are propped up on her desk. She measures my glasses in a machine that instantly produces my prescription in red crystal diode numerals.

I sit bleary-eyed in the waiting room, and wait for the drops to take effect. In fifteen minutes I am summoned back to her office.

She shines the light directly into my left eye. I look back and the veins of my eye resemble the canals of Mars. "Look up. Now to the upper right. Now to the right. Now to the lower right. Look down. Now to the lower left. Look left. Now to the upper left. Good." She clicks the lens machine, and now my left eye stares into blackness, and my right eye is exposed. I wonder whether she is interrogating me or the virus.

I hop onto the subway after my grossly extended lunch. Back at the office, I turn out all the lights. Even the CRT burns at its dimmest setting. After a few senseless hours, I blunder my way home.

Six months later, I return for my second appointment, but later in the day. Again, I forget my shades.

The receptionist hands me the clipboard. Any new drugs since the last visit? Change of address? I list them all, including my new allergies. It won't be long before my chart here is as voluminous as a novel by Trollope.

Dr. Judith evinces a mild interest that I find slightly patronizing. "Oh, you have that new book on gays and the military. Is it as good as the *Times* said yesterday?"

"I've only just started it."

After she gives me eye drops, she tells me I can read if I hold the book directly in front of my eyes without glasses. I sit and watch the room slowly grow blurry and bright, a fish inside a large bowl made of prescription-strength glass.

Briefly apologizing, she takes a personal phone call in the middle of my examination. Her husband can't find her son at the airport.

She examines my eyes through a monstrous magnifying glass I dub the Pupil Enlarger: a fifties horror sci-fi movie prop used to examine mutant flies and crabs exposed to radioactivity. With the calm patience of an affectless serial killer, she scrutinizes the blood vessels in my eyes.

"Your eyes aren't any worse. They're as bad as ever. Stay out of trouble. Have an uneventful six months."

I've forgotten to ask her about intravitreal implants.

I've had bad eyes since I was seven. I bet a friend at Day Camp Iroquois the unthinkable sum of a dollar that the arrow he had shot at the archery range was in the yellow. It was, in fact, in the blue ring. Shortly thereafter I got my first pair of glasses, to be replaced, each year, by a thicker model. With each new prescription the world suddenly presented itself to me with stunning clarity. I could actually see each individual blade of grass, each strand of carpet. Yes, this is the unexpected explanation for why nerds with glasses stare at their feet: We are continually astounded at our surroundings.

My eyesight grew so bad that for several years an ophthalmologist would give me drops, under the mistaken belief that the untouched eye would grow stronger to compensate for the weaker one. I remember weaving my way to the bus stop and missing the first two buses because the glaring light made it impossible to read the sign on the bus. Where is that fucking seeing-eye dog when you need him?

By twenty I was pathologically myopic. A barn would make a nice reference point if it didn't blur into dusk at ten feet. At the beach, after I gingerly removed my glasses, someone would have to point me in the direction of the ocean. After a brief dip at Venice Beach, I spent a good twenty minutes trying to find my towel, aided only by my friend Greg's raucous laughter.

I can't focus without my glasses. I lose my balance. Words become indistinct. Shouts become murmurs. All is in shadow.

I was raised on standardized multiple-choice aptitude tests. I remember working my way through the colored reading folders in sixth grade, going all the way up to gold. At eye exams I was in a constant state of anxiety: Am I answering correctly? Is the green letter really clearer than the red one? What do you do when the lenses flip into place and you can't distinguish? What happens if your left eye waters at that crucial moment? There are no study guides. There is no Stanley Kaplan crash course. Still, it was hard to avoid memorizing the eye chart on the wall moments before the questions would begin. I was always afraid that I would give the wrong answer and no one would know.

I've felt this way for doctors' exams. Am I remembering the correct symptoms? Am I asking all the correct questions? Is it a phantom pain in my feet or an actual neuropathic disorder? What is the exact quality of pain, mercy, fear, and hope?

After my examination, I reflect on how much my life revolves around seeing. I write on my laptop. For relaxation I read, or I go to a movie or a play. Everything I do is visual. What do I enjoy that doesn't involve my eyes? Sleep. There is only sleep.

What would I do if I became blind?

I would get a Kurzweil reader.

I would learn to appreciate music, which used to be nonvisual, before the advent of music videos.

I would have the microwave embossed with instructions in Braille.

I would learn Japanese from tapes.

I would get a Soloflex, because although as a person without sight I would have finally attained enough attitude to go to the gym, I would no longer be able to cruise, which effectively negates all justification to go.

I would try to remain self-sufficient: Perhaps I could install a vending machine in my apartment with cheese and crackers, peanut butter and crackers, macaroni and beef—that sort of thing. Each time I'd press the button, a new surprise would topple down.

I would move to an apartment with no view.

I would order out a lot.

I would only call numbers preprogrammed on my phone.

I would hire hustlers.

But ultimately what's the point in planning for contingencies?

Raul chided me when he found out I didn't have a comprehensive disability package. "You're not likely to get insurance now at any price," he told me. Raul was very well prepared. It was only natural. He worked for a gay investment firm. Raul had extensive insurance for disability that would have lasted for years.

Yet for all his planning and foresight, Raul was still dead in three months when KS ate away his lungs.

How to Visit Someone in the Hospital with a Terminal Disease

1. Bring gifts suitable to his disability. Don't bring a cassette of his favorite Audrey Hepburn movie if he's recently gone blind. Try to stay within his field of vision, if he has any left.

2. Remember to bring vases with flowers. He may need that plastic container for other, more urgent purposes: urine, for example.

3. Don't be offended if he falls asleep in the middle of your running commentary about your pet's crazy antics or your boss's latest tantrum: This may not have anything to do with his level of interest.

4. It may not be the best time to show him your latest piercing if he has just had a catheter implanted in his chest.

5. It may not be in the best of taste to brag about the fifth-row tickets you scored to Bette Midler by waiting in line for seven hours if the concert is next fall and he may not be around to read the reviews.

6. Don't feel compelled to share your recent rediscovery of God in the form of a Peruvian bodybuilder-masseur, unless, of course, you have explicit photos.

7. Don't take advantage of a captive audience: If he is hooked

up to an IV and life support, he may not especially want to hear your forty-two-act existential drama about the history of tobacco narrated through the viewpoint of a low-tar cigarette.

8. It is considered in poor taste to snip a lock of hair from his head, especially if you plan on incorporating it in a Guatemalan Santeria voodoo ceremony involving scattering chicken bones on the floor.

9. If his lover indicates that they would like some time alone, leave discreetly. Avoid giving blowjobs during doctors' rounds. Be considerate to his roommate. Remember to pull the curtains closed during intimate acts. Consider a discreet handjob as reparation for a minor disturbance.

10. A variety of magazines with photos is appropriate. The novels of Thomas Mann and Fyodor Dostoevsky are not. *The Magic Mountain* is the worst book to read when recovering from PC; Roth's *The Anatomy Lesson* is particularly inappropriate following a spinal tap.

11. Listen to what he says. Kiss him on the cheek. Touch him. Hold him. Rub his back. Massage his feet. Hold his hands. Look into his eyes. Feed him dinner. Wash his forehead. Wipe the sweat off his arms. Hold his hand while he receives an injection. Consider your hospital visit a field experiment for your personal course in self-assertiveness. Give the floor nurse hell for not changing the sheets. Scream at the resident when the painkiller doesn't arrive in time.

12. If, on the other hand, he was an enemy and made your life a living hell for the past five years, do take every opportunity to visit him in the hospital and feel free to perform any of the above contraindicated acts. You needn't do anything. Your mere presence at his inexorable decline should be enough.

Memorials from Hell

The invitation was tasteful and plain, a white card with no photograph: "A memorial service will be held for Paul Taylor [hyphenated years in brackets] on such-and-such date at 5:30 P. M. A short reception will follow." The address was that of a fashionable Soho gallery space. The envelope was stamped with a man's name and Paul's familiar address: I assume he was Paul's last lover. I suppose I dreaded the reception more than the service. For some reason, I was compelled to go, as if I had been summoned.

I knew Paul was positive, but I hadn't realized he was ill until I read his obituary in *The New York Times*.

No photos of Paul greeted me at the entrance. I'm sure this was a deliberate choice. Avedon's too expensive and Mapplethorpe's dead. I wonder what photo I would use: an embarrassing nude? But I suppose the point of memorials is not to humiliate those who come.

I came a bit too early: ten minutes before the ceremony was scheduled to start. People were clustering in small groups, trying to find those they knew. No one had sat down yet. I know this is

Originally appeared in Gay Community News, *April 1993.*

the height of hypocrisy, but please do not invite tricks and one-night-stands to my memorial. There is something sad about single men with sideburns sitting in scattered seats as if at an afternoon showing of some obscure Deanna Durbin movie. I can imagine myself at home, dragging my IV behind into my office, tossing out inappropriate names from my Rolodex in a frenzied fit. Should I code names in my address book with colored markers? I'm such a control queen, I just might write out the invitations myself in my hospital bed, surrounded by life-support equipment. And when the battery of my laptop needs recharging, relying on my friend who has medical power of attorney to help me decide which device to unplug: the portable television, the oxygen, or the respirator. I would probably write the reminiscences myself if I thought I could get away with it.

We've all been to memorials when the slightest of acquaintances testifies with a personal recollection. I just think it would be in poor taste for someone I had met on a phone-sex line to speak: "I knew him as Fred."

At weddings, sections are designated for friends and family of the groom and the bride. Memorials could divide seats into couples and singles to facilitate cruising. One-night-stands could sit at the back, near the hors d'oeuvres. A woman sitting in front of me said hi. I had no idea who she was.

Luckily I ran into my friend Jay, who sits next to me. Jay, it develops, had had a two-week affair with Paul; I had had a three-week affair. Jay had borrowed someone else's invitation; I received mine in the mail. I guess three weeks was the cutoff date. Paul dumped Jay because he was too fat; Paul dumped me because he was an empress and I was only a pitiful princess.

Nervously, I take out some Certs stored in a Ziploc storage bag in my backpack. Jay thought it was a drug. "Fifteen dollars from the PWA Health Group; I think they import it from Sweden. I can't wait until they get FDA approval; the cost is astronomical."

Paul had mastered the art of rudeness. He was brilliant. He was compelling. He had an incredible amount of personal charisma. He was not unlike Hitler. His friends loved him and were intensely loyal to him. His discards avoided him like the plague. He liked having me come over to his apartment for lunch so he could be continually interrupted by phone calls. He criticized my table manners because I didn't point my silverwear down in the European manner; I used the savage American style with fork tines up, although I don't understand the consistency of this approach given gravity and the tendency of soup to return to the bowl when the spoon is facing down.

Paul was quite simply a genius. His friends were devoted to him, and his former friends loathed him. Paul was a textbook example of the Squeeze song "If I Didn't Love You, I'd Hate You." He was the type of person whom you would never expect to die. Let's face it, some people you expect will die. With others you are shocked. I wasn't surprised when I read about Anthony Perkins having AIDS. The *Enquirer* never lies. After seeing *Crimes of Passion* I believed he was capable of anything.

Four women and one man addressed the crowd, leading one to wonder whether he had any male friends save the odd executor. Astonishingly enough, most of them mentioned Paul's rudeness during their speeches. One said she was surprised to find out Paul's age from the *Times* obituary; he had always led her to believe he was older. All the speakers were incredibly eloquent, so eloquent that they all elicited applause one might expect at a Broadway memorial. Of course, it would have been rude to greet subsequent speakers with silence after the first. Is it appropriate to applaud the cleverness of a speaker at a memorial service? Would Paul have approved? I doubt it. I still recall my ninth-grade choir teacher, who stopped the evening performance dead in its tracks to glare at the parents in the audience who dared applaud between movements. I have since relented in the silly judgment that under these circumstances clapping is boorish. The only boorish behavior would be to leave at the end of the ceremony, skipping the reception. In my private tribute to Paul, I left posthaste.

• • •

I had been overwhelmed by life. There were just too many things to do. Somehow I hadn't gotten around to visiting David and Luis. David Serko was a peripheral friend-of-a-friend whom I knew only remotely: enough to say hello to at the gym or at ACT UP. I was hoping to visit him with my friend Wayne.

Tom advised me against seeing Luis because he was doing so poorly. Perhaps Tom was overcompensating for asking me to visit his friend Charles after promising Charles I would see him. Tom shared a lot of his difficulties in dealing with Charles, and since they were such close friends, he rarely mentioned the good; consequently, I had an extremely poor opinion of Charles and was reluctant to visit. Hospital visits require an enormous amount of emotional energy: I feel they should be done selectively. Still, I knew Luis's lover, Jon, and however bad Luis was, I could always comfort Jon.

So I added "visit David and Luis" to my "to do" list on Sunday night. On Monday at noon I found out that David had died that morning. With double my determination, I went to see Luis that afternoon, after work. One hospital information person referred me to another; the second told me that Luis "had expired" yesterday. He had expired. Like a library book.

When I heard that Tom Cunningham had died, my first impulse was to call a friend and find out where he was when he heard; what he was doing; what he was thinking; how he was situated in time and space. Somehow I needed to share this. I want my death to be unforgettable, a bullet lodged in the spine, a scaly burr stuck in the neck, an alien organic presence that merges with its host and becomes a part of it, a virus that grows to overwhelm and kill, but then it would kill the memory: Death is the end of memory.

Several years ago some members of ACT UP would go leafleting on Sunday afternoons at Jones Beach and Fire Island. They were

given the nickname the Swim Team. God knows how many stories from *Honcho* and *Playguy* centered on the archetypal golden
boy from the high-school swim team. David Serko was the archetypal Swim Team member. Back in the early trendy days of ACT
UP, activism was sexy: At this moment it is in an off-cycle of wan-
ing popularity. I'm sure more than a few people went to ACT UP
meetings just to bask in David's beauty.

David was always pleasant to me. I was hoping to see him last
summer on Fire Island, when I rented a week at Wayne's house.
Unfortunately, he wasn't feeling well enough to travel then. He
was blind then.

I went to the memorial with Wayne. It was a church on 110th
Street, complete with organ, chorus, and fey minister. Out of respect for those who organized the service, I took a red ribbon and
impaled it on my jacket. Wayne didn't. The music reminded me
of a bad daytime soap opera. Our friend Ron told how David was
a bus captain for the Kennebunkport demonstration, and how he
quietly administered his one-hour drip of DHPG on the bus ride
up. People applauded after various speakers because they were expected to: David had, after all, toured Europe in *A Chorus Line.* I
stood when everyone else stood for a religious moment. Wayne
remained seated.

The service lasted three hours. *Angels in America* was quoted,
even though it hadn't yet opened in New York. Afterward I
rushed to a Publishing Triangle party, where I was chastised by another cynic for wearing a red ribbon.

I vowed that my service would be different. Guests would be
told that in the last few months of my life I became deeply interested in worshipping Satan. Instead of handing out red ribbons,
ushers would be instructed to write "666" in charcoal on the
foreheads of the guests. There might be a pagan sacrifice of a baby
lamb. Instead of an organ, there would be a kazoo. Oh, and Liza
has to sing "But the World Goes Round."

If David's memorial was the *Nicholas Nickleby* of memorials, my memorial would be a Ring Cycle marathon. My friend Michael Morrissey told me that he had topped me; his memorial was to be a subscription series.

Don't die in late November or December: Scheduling the memorial service will be hell. In addition to seasonal shopping, holiday parties, last-minute tax-deductible benefits, Stop the Church anniversary demos, and outlaw sex parties, you'll have to contend with Seasonal Affective Disorder. My friend Jan color-codes events in his datebook: December is a kaleidoscopic blur of stacked events. I had to go to a seasonal party and a birthday party after Luis's memorial, which started promptly Latino/Latina time an hour after it was scheduled to. Was I out of my fucking mind? It made no sense.

Luis's memorial was at the Manhattan Center for Living, a million psychic miles from the Frank Campbell Funeral Home. People were encouraged to come in drag. I had thought this was only for the lip-syncing performers: I stuck to the traditional black jeans and black-leather jacket. Luis was totally outrageous, and his memorial service was completely over the top. My friend Tom "channeled" Stevie Nicks wearing four skirts, black stockings, a cowl, and what seemed like three feet of teased blond hair, dancing like a lunatic. He then proceeded to strip to his jockstrap while telling a poignant tale of how he woke after an emergency appendectomy to Luis playing with his nipples and fainted as he saw his blanched father sitting at the base of the hospital bed. Heidi danced in leather chaps over pink panties. Jon, the widow, dressed in widow's weeds replete with black veil, did a lip-synced duet to Natalie and Nat Cole's "Unforgettable" with a posterboard photo of Luis that had a hinged manipulable mouth.

The Manhattan Center for Living follows the Marianne Williamson approach to illness. At one point in the memorial Jon read a letter that Luis had written to his illness, and the illness's reply. Absurdly, in this age of AIDS, Luis had leukemia. Luis had quit dancing professionally to become a full-time AIDS activist. I first met him in Atlanta, where he had flown for a series of ACT UP demonstrations to repeal the sodomy law and change the CDC definition of AIDS. Luis was an extraordinarily sexy man, filled with a tremendous capacity for joy and endless delight. There is no justice when someone like Luis has to die at twenty-seven. How can there possibly be a God, with leukemia and AIDS?

If some sadistic spiritualist forced me to write a letter to my illness, I think the exchange would go like this:

Dear HIV: Fuck you! I wish you were dead so I could live a normal life. I am terrified of dying. Yours in hell, David.

Dear David: Now, why don't you just be mature and adopt a New Age view and learn to accept me? Your faithful retrovirus, HIV.

Dear HIV: As John Weir once said when I asked him if he had slept with a woman, never never never never never never never never never never never.

The title of this piece is redundant. All memorials are Memorials from Hell.

How to Make a Will

Consider the fundamental rule of wills: Just because you are dead doesn't mean you have to cease being a control queen. Follow these simple rules and you, too, can wreak havoc from the grave.

1. Procrastinate for several years.

2. Enumerate all your worldly possessions. Include any item valued at more than five books of S&H green stamps. Certain mementos of solely sentimental value (unsigned *Playbills*, calculus textbooks, and those loose slips of paper with first name and number, for example) should be listed separately.

3. Make a list of your friends. When you are done with your will, you can revise it monthly. This will keep your friends on their toes.

4. Make a list of your enemies. *Don't leave them out.* By remembering them in your will, you will be able to get back at them from beyond the grave. For example, it could be a nice gesture to deed a double-headed dildo to an enemy who is an ostensible top, especially if the will is to be read in public.

5. Nude photographs and other suggestive material should be

distributed to friends before you are dead. Families have a tendency to destroy these things inadvertently.

6. The condoms have probably expired by now, so you might as well throw them out.

7. Instruct your executor to burn your unfinished manuscripts, musical-comedy scores, and dress designs. There is nothing more embarrassing than having some hack complete your final symphony. You are responsible for your reputation, shoddy as it may be. Don't risk having it ruined by someone else.

8. Remember your favorite charities. Consider, for example, endowing an especially uncomfortable chair in sadomasochism for the Center for Lesbian and Gay Studies at CUNY grad school.

9. You are capable of causing mischief from the urn. Divide an item between two people who passionately dislike each other, forcing them to bargain. For example, give Bertram the frame of your favorite Eames chair and give Maurice, his ex, the seat.

10. Be very careful to whom you plan on giving your black book.

11. Think about distributing your ashes in acrylic paperweights and giving them to your friends and/or enemies. This would serve as a constant reminder of your presence. These items are particularly difficult to throw away or sell at rummage sales.

Everything
You Do Is
Wrong

When I told Barry in January 1993 that I was down to 90 T-cells, but I was okay about it—I wasn't hysterical, as I was last year when I dropped below 100 once—he said, "Why aren't you?" So, of course, I immediately became hysterical. This wasn't your traditional standing-on-the-tabletop-pulling-your-hair-and-screaming-at-the-top-of-your-lungs hysterical: I like to think of it as a persistent low-grade hysteria, like a persistent low-grade fever. With me it's more internal: screaming voices that only I can hear; looking into the bathroom mirror and seeing portions of my face collapse and fall off like dirt into the sink, until I resemble Alexis Smith on the poster for Sondheim's *Follies* or Mount Rushmore being sandblasted.

The key to understanding me or anyone else who's HIV-positive is simple: Everything you do is wrong. My boss passed on an article from the *Miami Herald* about some drug trial in Florida that her boss's former colleague was involved in. "I thought you might be interested in this," she wrote on the yellow sticker. A thirty-six-year-old former hairdresser was undergoing infusion therapy. He complained that he would have to lie down and take a nap for a few hours after the gym. He didn't look half bad. I am exactly thirty-six, go to the gym constantly, and could easily pass for a former hairdresser with my new Vanessa-Redgrave-in-*Playing-for-Time* hairstyle. Was this one similarity too many?

I appreciated her interest and concern. The problem was that my boss had given me this during the twenty minutes of the day that I wasn't thinking about AIDS.

Like most HIV-positive people, I spend 95 percent of my waking hours thinking about AIDS. Here is a breakdown of the thought processes of an average gay man in his mid-thirties (note that percentages add up to considerably more than 100 percent, because I am capable of worrying about as many as five things simultaneously):

95 percent: AIDS. Has the wart or mole on my cheek changed? Is that cough a precursor to PCP? Is my upset stomach a sign of gastrointestinal CMV? Is the tingly feeling in my hands and feet worsening? Are my gums bleeding again? Am I sleeping enough? Am I sleeping too much? Am I more tired than I was a week ago? Am I seeing floaters? Is my vision impaired, or do I just need to clean my glasses? Am I having trouble hearing, or do I just have a gob of ear wax in my left ear? Do I have an appropriate outfit for the memorial service this Thursday?

80 percent: Sex. Is the guy whose personal ad in *Homo Xtra* I answered two and a half weeks ago going to call me when my extremely jealous boyfriend is here? Is the cute boy at the gym who used to wear leopard-skin Lycra shorts and who's turning thirty this March and who made me do fifteen minutes of abdominal exercises with him ever going to finish his workout and take a shower? If you stare at the bulge in a Marky Mark underwear poster long enough, will you fall into it? Does Madonna ever have lesbian sex with men in drag? Which movie star is Jodie Foster's rumored love interest? If Brad Pitt's film career crashes, will he ever be leading ab classes at the Chelsea Gym? Is there a gym remote enough in Manhattan for me to escape my hideous past? If

all my former boyfriends got together, would there be a catfight or an orgy? Who is my next prospective former boyfriend? Do I have an appropriate outfit for the sex party this Sunday?

48 percent: Food. Should I try some new American Lean Cuisine tonight or stick with Thai takeout or something from the gourmet deli around the corner? Am I going to end up like Goldie Hawn in *Death Becomes Her*, eating frosting directly from the can? Has anyone ever in recorded history kept a box of Pepperidge Farm cookies for longer than three days? Why are all my boyfriends vegetarian?

25 percent: Madonna. Has Madonna done enough for the AIDS crisis? How did my mother know that I would buy a copy of *Sex* the day it was released? Is Madonna ever going to have a viable film career? Is the reason that *Erotica* didn't include printed lyrics their sheer banality? How many magazines is Madonna going to be on the cover of in 1993? What's Madonna's next look? What will Madonna look like at fifty? Am I changing my physical appearance and reinventing myself as often as Madonna?

18 percent: What would Bette Davis say in this situation?

0 percent: What's on television tonight?

If you ask me how I'm feeling, I'll feel that you're invading my privacy, giving me the third degree, bringing up a topic that I don't particularly wish to discuss at the present time. But if you don't ask me, I'll feel neglected, unwanted, denied any empathy. You can't win. Everything you do is wrong.

Paradoxically, now that I understand this, it matters less. I can hardly get angry when I know in advance that whatever anyone does it will undoubtedly be wrong. Despite the best of intentions, no one will ever get it.

So when Binky asks me, "How are you feeling?"

I tell him, "I'm feeling fine."

"Are you sure?" he persists.

"I'm fine."

"Are there any changes in your symptoms since last week?" he inquires.

"What symptoms?" I ask myself. "No," I tell him.

"Are you sure?" he inquires.

At wit's end, I admit, "I'm getting a headache." Probably from this exchange, I mutter beneath my breath.

"I'm so sorry," he allows.

And then I have a seizure and blurt out, "I might as well tell you that yes, I got PCP while you were away, but I've completely recovered and I would have told you earlier if it hadn't slipped my mind or what's left of it from my dementia."

Finally satisfied, he gives me a bemused smile and returns to *The New York Times* crossword puzzle, contentedly filling in the squares with letters in ink.

Miss Letitia Thing's New Guide to Excruciatingly Correct Behavior for the Dying

1. Use your discretion to determine whether you wish to receive an audience. Try not to be too irritated should a visitor bring an inappropriate favor. Resist the impulse to criticize their appearance. This is a trying time for both of you.

2. Take all the medication you want. Clarity isn't always necessary at this point.

3. Don't feel guilty about the sudden need or desire for a priest or reverend, even if you've been brought up as an orthodox Jew.

4. It's all right to act a little spoiled. This may be your last chance to be a prima donna. Make the most of it.

5. Feel free to invent extravagant chores so those less-amusing acquaintances can feel useful. If you have a sudden craving for toasted-coconut donuts from the South Bronx, I'm sure you can assign this task to the appropriate visitor.

6. Tell your friends if you want to be alone. Don't feel obligated to entertain them into exhaustion. If they don't know how to amuse themselves without you, they'd better start practicing.

7. Ask for what you need. This may seem obvious, but it is very difficult for most people. Do not be disappointed if a simple request isn't fulfilled. Instead, consider revising your will.

8. Short-term memory problems may result from either the drugs you are taking or those pesky neurological difficulties. Don't feel embarrassed asking the strangers who visit what their names are. If one responds "Dad," kindly pat his hands and tell him you were merely performing a psychological test on him and he passed, even if he still looks rather unfamiliar.

9. Don't be afraid of the tunnel of white light. It's just a special effect designed by George Lucas's Industrial Light and Magic Company; it has something to do with that computer chip they soldered into your brain the last time they put you under. It is intended to comfort you when the time comes.

10. Don't feel guilty about overstaying your welcome. Until we have universal health care and a single-payer system, you will be merely bilking some insurance company that has raped thousands over and over again. It is, in fact, your civic duty to run up the highest hospital bill. Pretend you are playing a pinball game, and your bill is your running score. Just keep on working at it and you may be allowed to enter your initials in the Book of Life.

A
Season
in Hell

I see my doctor a lot these days. We have this ongoing relationship. Today I'm here because there's a tickle in my throat that may or may not be strep. Also, it's time to get weighed and go over possible symptoms and have blood drawn to check my T-cell and platelet counts and various antibody and antigen levels, and to get a shot of B_{12} and a shot of pentamidine and get refills for my prescriptions that have run out since my last visit four weeks ago. *Don't even think of mentioning managed care to me.*

You see, I have AIDS. Sometimes I find it difficult to tell people I am gay; coming out as a person with AIDS can be even more complicated. Do you tell everyone, including your boss at work, who recently slapped you with a rather poor annual review? Do you tell only your closest friends and the people whom you've had intimate knowledge of in the past fifteen years? Is there a difference? When you are introduced to a prospective former-boyfriend or a potential lifelong friend, is it appropriate to say, "Hi, my name is Dave. I'm gay and I have AIDS. Pleased to meet you"? The only time I feel comfortable not disclosing my

Originally appeared as "HIV + Me" in Details, January 1994.

serostatus is during phone sex, but I still feel guilty faking orgasms. I figured that coming out in *Details* would save a lot of agonizing phone calls and postage stamps.

I officially got my AIDS diagnosis on New Year's Day 1993. I knew in advance this would happen and there was absolutely nothing I could do about it. Recall the classic photo of Harold Lloyd dangling from a clock, hanging on for dear life? Imagine me up there, hopelessly attempting to stop time. I could blow up the ball that drops in Times Square at the stroke of midnight; I could hijack a Lear jet to travel endlessly through the International Date Line. Alternatively, I could make it appear that time had stopped or slowed down to an imperceptible rate by reading Michel Foucault or calling Time-Warner cable and being put on hold for half an hour. But all these solutions would only forestall the inevitable.

I'm not ready to be called a PWA yet. The phrase "AIDS victim" is definitely not chic. "AIDS patient" is inaccurate, because I'm hardly spending most of my time in the hospital. There must be *some* acronym that accurately conveys my anxiety and despair.

I hold the Centers for Disease Control and Prevention responsible for my predicament. I've been HIV-positive for more than a decade, but as yet I have had no major health problems; most of my difficulties have been related to bad reactions to prophylactic drugs. But my T-cells have been lower than 200 for more than a year now. Effective January 1, 1993, the CDC revised the definition of AIDS, adding a few new opportunistic infections and cervical cancer to the list; it also added the surrogate marker of fewer than 200 T-cells.

Getting AIDS was like turning thirty: The anticipation was horrible, but the actual event turned out to be a nonevent. With my brand-new AIDS diagnosis, I could conceivably go on disability and become a full-time AIDS activist, but I fear my health care would suffer. I'm somewhat addicted to my current doctor and my current health insurance.

There's something very Sylvia Plath about dreading the decades. After I turned twenty there was an adolescent suicide-attempt (an overdose of Flintstone vitamins: I paced through the drugstore for hours, but couldn't find the nonprescription sleeping pills). And now I want nothing more than to live to forty. My father died at fifty-two of his first heart attack, so, somewhat superstitiously, that age seems to be an absolute limit. At least it *was,* before I knew I was infected with HIV.

I remain a thirty-six-year-old gay white male with AIDS, formerly on the cusp of the epidemic, now fleeing the demographics. As the rate of infection lowers for gay men, more and more women, injection-drug users, and people of color are getting infected. This is undoubtedly due to the adoption of safer-sex practices among gay men; also, the virus has saturated the gay community. An estimated 50 percent of gay men in New York City and San Francisco are HIV-positive. AIDS has become a growth industry. I counted eight ads from viatical settlement companies in a recent issue of *The Advocate.* These companies buy life insurance from the terminally ill: the shorter your life expectancy, the better your return on investment. Then there's LifeStyle Urns™, which offers quality cremation urns with a lambda etched on the lid. They run from $249 to $349, with an optional velvet lining for $18 extra, if you supply the material. I guess that's to stop the bones from rattling.

My doctor takes a throat culture. I've had intermittent sore throats and been mildly fatigued for so long that I honestly don't know what "normal" is. My doctor gives me a prescription for rifabutin to prevent MAI, an opportunistic infection similar to tuberculosis that typically strikes those with fewer than 50 T-cells. Today I am down to 84. My doctor says it might also work for my sore throat. In any event, it will turn my pee orange.

He also injects my left hand with alpha interferon to try to cure my warts. He does this directly into nine separate warts with a needle I find a bit too large. I daub with cotton as he continues to pierce me. By the time the process is over, my hand resembles Saint Sebastian's. My doctor warns me that I may feel flulike side effects from the alpha interferon.

I never expected to be an expert on medical matters, and I still struggle. Now terms like "surrogate markers" and "nucleoside analogue" and "proteinase inhibitor" run trippingly off my tongue as easily as "slate-gray tile" and "track lighting." I try to keep informed. I'm buried in information that I don't have the time to read. I subscribe to GMHC's *Treatment Issues,* John James's *AIDS Treatment News,* Project Inform's *PI Perspective,* the PWA Health Group's *Notes from the Underground,* San Francisco AIDS Foundation's *Bulletin of Experimental Treatments for AIDS,* and the AmFAR *AIDS/NIV Treatment Directory,* and I pick up ACT UP's *Treatment and Data Digest* at the meetings. I usually pick up the PWAC NY *Newsline* and *The Body Positive* at the bookstore. Taking care of yourself is a full-time job.

Andrew Holleran wrote that the only news we are waiting for is the article on the front page of *The New York Times* titled "Cure Found." Well, last winter the *Times* announced the latest cure on the front page and I didn't even clip it. This approach was called convergent therapy: In a test tube, AZT, ddI, and pyridinone were able to completely stop the replication of HIV. The theory was that each drug would target viral mutations resistant to the others. Then again, according to Sally Cooper of the PWA Health Group, *gasoline* kills HIV in the test tube. No doubt some people will read this and roam through underground parking lots, lurking in the shadows, sniffing exhaust pipes.

I've seen enough "Cures of the Month" going down like lead balloons in the past few years. There are the vampire approaches, where blood products from virgins or people who didn't sleep around that much are introduced into the body, or extracorporeal hypothermia, where blood is drained and heated, then returned to the body. Ozone and herbal mixtures may be introduced through the orifice of your choice—my own personal favorite is bitter-melon enemas. Megadosing with vitamins such as beta carotene gives one an unhealthy orange glow and will probably be a fashionable look in some future century. I still remember that historic day when Larry Kramer himself announced the end of the epidemic, courtesy of compound Q, on the floor of a Monday-night ACT UP meeting.

Everyone responds differently to HIV infection. Some people change diets. Some join support groups. For me, ACT UP functions as a support group and a means of achieving change. I am personally skeptical of natural and holistic treatments. I am an atheist, after all. Later, when I'm down to 3 T-cells and about to have a deathbed conversion, I'm sure I'll eat all the kelp I can keep down. I believe in taking vitamins, but I feel that megadoses will either flush through the system or poison it. Alternative and holistic treatments work for people who have faith in them. I am so skeptical I lay most of their efficacy on the placebo effect: I prefer Tic Tacs or Toblerones. Acupuncture, massage, herbal treatments, and aromatherapy probably enhance the immune system by reducing stress. We're all waiting for some magical cure made of natural substances that has no toxicity. Unfortunately, it probably doesn't exist.

Ten years ago I was tired of my obsession with being gay. The prospect of undergoing the exhaustive promiscuous sex necessary to retain my status according to Kinsey overwhelmed me. A little voice inside me was constantly reminding me that I was different and that I could hide this from the world if I chose and that I could deny it to myself, but no matter what I did I would always be different. Eventually I adjusted. I am still adjusting to AIDS.

I'm sick and tired of thinking about AIDS all the time. I'm simultaneously obsessed and repelled by the idea of AIDS. I would like to take a vacation from AIDS. (In Biarritz? Tunisia? Perhaps Uruguay?) I would like to spend just one day not thinking about

AIDS at all, but the necessity of taking certain medications several times a day forces me to confront it daily.

Each day I take three capsules of AZT, along with six Zovirax, three Trental, two multiple antioxidant vitamins, one lysine tablet, and one aspirin. AZT is a nucleoside analogue that interferes with the synthesis of reverse transcriptase; thus, it inhibits the replication of HIV. Researchers believe it is effective against HIV for up to eighteen months, and I've been taking it for three years. There are problems with toxicity and resistant strains of the mutating virus. Zovirax is an antiviral that targets the herpes virus. I'm pretty sure Zovirax is working. I haven't had an outbreak in years. Herpes can act synergistically with HIV. My friend Glenn Pumilia experimented with stopping Zovirax, and his herpes came back virulently. He died on July 4, 1991.

I like Trental because it's pink. Trental is another drug that may or may not work. It is a blood viscosity remover used to treat painful leg cramps associated with arteriosclerotic disease. My doctor prescribes it off-label because research indicates it may inhibit HIV in the test tube. I also take two antioxidant vitamins, the most expensive vitamin I have ever bought, sixty dollars for 250 pills. And lysine, an amino acid that suppresses herpes. And a tablet of aspirin. My friend Michael Morrissey was taking aspirin daily and it did wonders for his T-cells. I didn't get the same effect, but then I was using Duane Reade generic and he was using Bayer.

After the doctor, I reward myself with an overpriced takeout lunch at the gourmet deli with the cute counterperson who has biceps the size of grapefruits. I generally go on sugar binges after dental visits, especially when I get root planing. I feel okay over the weekend, maybe a little weaker than usual. On Tuesday I am so exhausted I stay home from work. My body aches all over and I have a severe headache. I feel better Wednesday. My doctor's partner leaves a message on voice mail at work; I call back to discover I have strep throat and Hemophilus, another common throat infection. I tell him I feel much better; maybe the rifabutin has cured it. Then at four I start shivering. I feel like going straight home, but I have to go to Tom Cunningham's memorial at five-thirty. It is January 27, 1993. Tom Cunningham was ACT UP's work-space manager for a year and a half, and he introduced me to the music of k. d. lang three years ago. We flirted together for several months. Then two years ago we had a violent disagreement about whether the Heritage of Pride Committee should have a special category of "Best AIDS Float" in the Gay and Lesbian Pride Parade. Tom was a tireless advocate for the rights of the disabled. He frequently interpreted meetings, concerts, and conferences for the hearing-impaired. I can't miss this service. I take another rifabutin.

Bob Rafsky speaks at Tom Cunningham's memorial. Bob is one of my biggest heroes. He went to a meeting with a Japanese pharmaceuticals company that was delaying work on a promising treatment for KS. Out of fury and frustration, he rolled up one of his pants legs and placed his lesion-covered leg on the table, a direct object lesson of his anger. I could only think of Nikita Khrushchev taking off his shoe and banging it on the table for attention at the U.N. Bob has challenged presidential candidate Clinton face to face to take action on the AIDS crisis: "You're dying of ambition. We're dying." The AP photo of them face to face was in every newspaper in the country.

In a way, Bob Rafsky is the heart and soul of ACT UP. Through his eloquent and passionate speeches, Bob can fire us up. He is ACT UP's unofficial cheerleader, always rousing us to attend the next rally or demonstration with a stirring call to action. Yet he is highly selective in his causes. Bob has the guts to cut through the crap and dismiss an irrelevant zap. "What does this have to do with saving lives? Why else are we here?" Bob Rafsky is our bravest warrior, and at the same time our ever-goading conscience.

Bob says that this is the last memorial at which he will ever speak. His endless eloquence always astounds me: It takes him longer to state his reasons for refusing to speak at another memorial than most other people's entire testimonies. But then again, I am cranky and shivering. I love Bob Rafksy. Bob refers to himself as the Kaposi's sarcoma poster child. He is obviously in pain. He says, "I feel that my speaking is also disrespectful because it flies in the face of the absoluteness of Tom's death and all the other deaths, as if in the face of that my words could give a sense of closure, of significance, of comfort. In fact, another AIDS death signifies nothing and there isn't or shouldn't be any comfort. So I've made a vow that this is the last memorial at which I will speak."

I bolt after the service and take a cab home.

People simply disappear. Obituaries are posted on the bulletin board at the gym next to Fire Island shares. I always wonder whether someone had just died when I see notices for furniture at drastically reduced rates. There comes a point when you realize you've gone to so many memorials that at the height of hubris you start thinking about your own, how to make it the craziest, the most memorable, the most outrageous—somehow forgetting that you won't be in attendance. You fear you're going to end up as a four-by-six section of cloth that keeps growing exponentially.

I'm sick and tired of red ribbons and the Names Quilt. There's something "nice" about a red ribbon for AIDS awareness. There's nothing "nice" about AIDS. Leave it to some design queens to transform a plague into a fashion statement. As for the Names Quilt, I don't want to end up a rectangular rag, however suitably decorated. The textile responses to the AIDS crisis leave me cold. I prefer to wear my ACT UP button that says "ACT UP, FIGHT BACK, FIGHT AIDS" and have people on the subway cringe when they read the last word on it.

I spend the next day in bed. I call my doctor again. He is on vacation, so his partner calls in a prescription to the local pharmacy for Augmentin for the strep throat. He doesn't want to give me something for the Hemophilus too because two antibiotics would do a number on my stomach. Somehow I deduce that I have been less ill from the strep throat than from side effects of the rifabutin. I stop the rifabutin and start Augmentin.

I have ten delightful days of Augmentin. It wipes me out. The only side effect of Augmentin is mild diarrhea, which Imodium A-D keeps under control. My sore throat improves. I take acidophilus to restore stomach bacteria that the penicillin is killing. Do I sound like your maiden great-aunt from Philadelphia? I think the pills may have gotten me depressed; then again, this could be my natural state.

The day after I finish Augmentin, I go to visit my friend Jim Lewis, who has just gotten out of the hospital. Jim has a host of problems. His KS is systemic, his stomach isn't working properly, and he's lost fifteen pounds in the past month; he's all teeth and bones. I go uptown to his apartment. I pick up the umbrella I had forgotten last May after GMHC's AIDS Walk. He and his lover had a housewarming that evening. It rained torrents last year that day; I dropped off my checks at the mud-filled fields of Central Park and ended up doing the AIDS Walk on the stair machine at the gym.

I try to avoid Jim's cat, who is particularly friendly. I became slightly allergic to cats when I turned thirty. Although I will deny it emphatically, I am increasingly sensitive. This has nothing to do with my sexual orientation.

I take the subway downtown for my affinity group's final meeting before the Hoffmann–La Roche demo. We are planning on shutting their plant down for the day by blocking all eleven gates. Hoffmann–La Roche has committed a multitude of sins as a pharmaceuticals company; it all boils down to greed. Our demands include an end to the delay in developing the tat inhibitor, a compound that, if effective, might actually kill HIV inside infected cells; the release of the data on European trials of a protease inhibitor; post-marketing studies on ddC, which was only provisionally approved; and a reduction in the price of the polymerase chain reaction, a genetic technology used to test for HIV infection.

I have been involved in planning this action for months. We are going to handcuff ourselves together inside metal pipes and block the entrances at 7:00 A.M. Visualize a chain of paper dolls that has been bronzed. I am hungry and our meeting isn't for another half hour so I stop and have an egg roll at a Chinese takeout on Second. The middle is still frozen.

At the meeting I feel flushed. My friend Tom tells me I have a rash. We practice hooking our handcuffs onto the bar inside the metal pipe and linking up together. We position ourselves as we would be inside the van on Tuesday morning. We pretend to jump out of a van's back door and link up into a solid barrier. I am tired and hot and sweaty. My rash is getting worse. After a few hours, I go home, exhausted. I am itchy all over.

Monday night after work I have a meeting with the board of the co-op that I have been trying to buy for several months. I go to work. I don't go to the doctor. I am taking Benadryl for my rash. I figure I have an allergic reaction to the cat or the egg roll. The rash is all over my body. I wonder whether I should postpone the co-op board meeting. My original loan will expire in one week; any delay involves the risk of a higher rate.

I am filled with misgivings. I have hated my rent-stabilized studio for close to thirteen years, but it's too cheap for me to leave it. It is a one-floor walk-up. When you are planning future disabilities, these things matter. Every Saturday from eleven at night to two in the morning I listen to the raucous sounds of salsa from the South American restaurant next door. My apartment is a large two-room studio, but since my boyfriend moved in, it feels even more cramped than before.

The rent would be manageable on public disability. Could I risk a move at 84 T-cells? Why should I buy when I could rent?

Would my estate be able to sell the apartment in a reasonable amount of time? Is there room for a respirator and a hospital bed? The building has an elevator, but there are five steps in front. How could I keep up with the mortgage and maintenance if I lost my job? Social Security goes only so far. What do I do if I run out of my retirement fund? Will I be forced to spend down to get on Medicare? Do they take away your apartment before you can qualify for public assistance? Why don't I rent a luxury apartment with a doorman and concierge services if I want to spend all my money now? What will my family do if they are stuck with an apartment in New York? How can I in good conscience spend the money I should be leaving them in my will when they live so frugally and the Fruit of the Month Club goes only so far?

But the real subtext is, "Have I started sliding down that slippery slope?"

I'm sure every HIV-positive person thinks this periodically. Minor aches and pains magnify in the mind's echo tunnel. Sure, it's just a minor cough, *now.* But suppose it's the start of the long decline. Suppose things only get worse. I generally get this feeling once a week. I have mild allergies, and sometimes I feel that my lung capacity is lower than normal, and I am convinced that I have PCP because maybe I fucked up inhaling pentamidine the last time at my crowded doctor's office when I ran into my friend Stewart downstairs. I felt as if we were sharing an ice-cream soda with two straws as the two of us puffed furiously. Will this free-floating anxiety ever leave me and float off into the stratosphere, where it belongs?

What will I do when I experience my first life-threatening symptoms? Will I lie to my doctor and stuff my pockets with rocks to camouflage weight loss? What will happen when I get diarrhea? My boyfriend pees a lot. Will I have to install a Portosan in the bedroom? Should I tell all my friends what my favorite foods are now that I am still coherent? What will happen when I can no longer metabolize chocolate? Is Godiva available in IV drips?

There are instructions in my will to shoot me if I ever get religion, because at that point I will have exhibited a complete loss of self.

I don't postpone the meeting with the co-op board. The members couldn't care less about my rash; they are interested only in my financials and whether or not I play a musical instrument. I forget to mention I have a boyfriend, Binky, who will be living with me.

My boyfriend is negative. Sometimes I feel like damaged goods. He has a fifty-year warrantee, and I'm stuck with a failed inspection slip in my shirt pocket: no refunds or exchanges, cash and carry only. I'm a time bomb waiting to go off. I'm an accident waiting to happen.

I have a friend Seth who is ten years younger than I am. I realize with some chagrin that I was probably getting infected during his Bar Mitzvah.

I read the Personals where people advertise for "healthy" people. I can't blame them. I wouldn't want to date someone with . . . gout. A lot of vegetarians don't date carnivores. Let's face it: We're all going to hell anyway. Some of us are just taking the express. Still, there is a certain amount of sexual apartheid going on. Just casually announce your antibody status at the next orgy and see how fast they all run for the showers. There is also an illogical psychological distinction made between performing certain sexual acts (specifically, oral sex without ejaculation) with someone who doesn't know his status and someone who does. The theory of safe sex says: Assume your partner is positive and act accordingly. In practice, many *hope* their partners are negative and act accordingly. I have been rejected after saying I was HIV-positive, but the absurd thing is that I am certain I've been rejected by someone who was also positive but didn't know because he hadn't taken the test.

There's a certain advantage to dating someone who is positive, if you are positive. You can share nebulizers, prescriptions, and possibly even urns. You can try pooling antibodies and T-cells. You don't have to worry about infecting each other; reinfection is only a Venial Sin, whereas initial infection is a Mortal Sin. Also, your partner won't run out screaming when you cut yourself shaving.

A few years ago I went to a PWA Coalition tea hosted by Michael Callen at the request of my friend John. I met Glenn Pumilia, who had come to keep his friend Frank company. Glenn and I dated for a few months. It would be nice to celebrate our anniversary with a toast in some seedy downtown cocktail lounge, but Glenn, John, and Frank are all dead. Michael Callen died in December 1993.

I sleep over at my friend Wayne's apartment that night because I can't face taking a taxi or a subway to our meeting Tuesday morning at 5:15 A.M. We are picking up demo supplies in the East Village and meeting our vans. I almost have enough clothes. It's hard to manipulate the handcuffs and clips wearing thick gloves. I bought thin white outdoor gloves from Paragon Sporting Goods Monday during lunch.

We demonstrate and freeze for two hours. Miraculously, we aren't arrested. The temperature is thirty-two. Anne comments that my face is still flushed from the cold. I realize it is my rash. I'm so itchy that night I can't get to sleep for hours. I end up taking two Ativans. On Wednesday I see my doctor, who tells me I am suffering from a delayed hypersensitive reaction to the Augmentin. He gives me a shot of cortisone. I am better for a few hours. I see him on Friday, because I still feel like shit. He prescribes prednisone as well as another antibiotic because I still have a throat infection.

So now I know I'm allergic to penicillin, in addition to sulfa drugs (which I tried a few years ago as PCP prophylaxis) and rifabutin. At this rate I will have sixty-three infections by the year 2000 and be able to tolerate only Sesame Street vitamins.

My mother calls me on Wednesday to tell me my grandmother is dying. She is ninety-four years old and lives in the Jewish Home for the Aged of Central New York. She has just gotten over her third bout of pneumonia. She has been senile for the past few years and isn't taking food. They could take her to a hospital and force-feed her, but that would probably extend her life for only a few weeks. It is only a matter of time.

My grandmother is semiconscious; she isn't responsive. There is no point in flying up to see her. I tell my mother I can't come up to say good-bye to my grandmother, but of course I will be there for the funeral. She starts crying. I can't believe I said the word *funeral* to my mother. I hang up.

My doctor calls me on Thursday to tell me to stop taking the drug I am taking and to start Ceftin. It turns out I still have Hemophilus, which isn't responsive to the drug he had prescribed. I thought he *knew* I had Hemophilus. His partner does. I have to keep on top of everything. It's difficult when you're not feeling well to do a proper job of monitoring your health care. I have to take ten days of Ceftin. Back to square one.

Friday morning my lawyer calls me to tell me that we are closing on Tuesday, the day the loan expires. He suggests I get co-op insurance. He tells me the amounts I need for certified or bank checks. I speed off to the bank and then to Allstate.

Monday is a holiday, Presidents' Day.

The closing takes place on Tuesday. I sleep badly the night before. "This is a mistake, this is a mistake, this is a mistake," is my sleeping mantra. The seller, the object of yet another one of my pathological flirtations, has troubles of his own. He flew in from San Francisco over the weekend because his mother is undergoing triple-bypass surgery. She is going under the knife as we sign a dozen documents. He hadn't slept at all the night before.

I use my ridiculous Bugs Bunny and Friends checks for the down payment. I decide if the sale ever goes through, my next set of checks will not contain rainbow flags, animated cartoon characters, or images of Judy Garland.

My mother tells me on Wednesday that my grandmother isn't doing any better. I realize that I haven't done my pentamidine in a month. I take pentamidine twice a month; once a month I inhale aerosol pentamidine in my doctor's office, and two weeks later he gives me a shot of pentamidine in the butt. I am planning on making an appointment to see my doctor on Friday, by which time I would be almost finished with the Ceftin. He could check my throat and give me my shots. But I decide to wait on making my appointment. I am anxious over my grandmother.

My grandmother dies on Thursday. I decide I will fly up early Friday morning. I spend Thursday evening in Bed Bath & Beyond with Binky, burying myself in a consumer frenzy to forget my larger reality. In an orgy of consumerism, we get queen-size sheets, pillowcases, and towels.

I have a tuxedo but no suit. My job is at a not-for-profit, which means I don't have to wear a tie. The only reason I would need a suit would be for job interviews, funerals, and co-op interviews. The tuxedo is for AIDS benefits.

Binky had borrowed my only nice long-sleeve white shirt. I have another one with coffee stains around the collar, which is odd, because I don't drink coffee. On Thursday night we have one of our typically passive-aggressive fights. Voices are never raised. In the aftermath of the fight, it is difficult to tell that a fight has taken place. The only telltale clue is that the cookbooks have been alphabetized; the silverware has been polished; and there is a dent the size of a human head in the plaster.

In a fit of controlled anger, Binky takes the shirt out of the laundry bag, washes it in Woolite in the sink, and hangs it on the shower rod to dry. He wakes up with me at 6:10 in the morning to iron it. I walk to Port Authority, take the bus to Newark, and ride the plane to Syracuse. My mother specified: no sneakers. I have my tight shoes in my garment bag.

I feel an enormous amount of guilt over my grandmother. I once wrote a fateful line in a story: "I wondered who would die first: me or my grandmother." It's one thing to exploit yourself in your fiction and another to exploit your own grandmother. And now I feel guilty writing about the circumstances of her death.

My sister and brother-in-law pick me up at the airport. My mother hasn't slept at all the night before. She won't sleep until my grandmother is buried. They are lucky to be able to arrange the funeral for Friday afternoon. If they can't do it by the evening, they will have to wait until Sunday, after the Jewish Sabbath.

My mother paces from room to room, dusting. She has no appetite. We make sandwiches and wait. She takes a bite of half a sandwich, then leaves the rest on the plate. "Don't eat too much, it's fifteen dollars a head for the buffet afterward," she warns. We are supposed to go to the funeral home at 1:00. Calling hours are from 1:30 to 2:30 P.M., which is when the funeral will start. My mother keeps peering through the front door She doesn't want to leave before her older sister. My aunt's car will go first in the procession.

My sister asks me if I would mind removing my earring. I ask her why. She says Mom asked her to ask me to remove it; she didn't want to ask me directly. This is how we communicate. It is important that I de-gay myself. Earrings still mean something in Syracuse, I suppose. I have an absolute fear of being in fashion. I generally wait five years after a trend has gone out of style before taking action. By the time I finally pierced my ear three years ago, models were piercing navels, singers were piercing cheeks, and in order to reside in the East Village one was required to have at least seven separate piercings.

The gold hoop takes forever to put in, even with a mirror. And then I need help connecting the loop. My next piercing will probably be a Hickman catheter in my chest so I can do daily delivery of ganciclovir to keep my CMV retinitis in check.

When I visit Syracuse I have to stifle myself. My conversation is reduced to an appropriate level of discourse: that of a precocious fifth-grader, or a severely retarded adult. I lose my mental acuity in Syracuse. Simple logistics become complicated. Conscious thought becomes difficult. Smothered by circumstance and surroundings, I stare blankly at the walls.

My sartorial anxieties turn out to be unfounded. I am the only one wearing a white shirt. Lonnie has a light-blue Oxford. My cousin Stan wears a plaid flannel shirt.

I've gone to so many memorials and funerals in the past few years that I have enough points of reference to rate this one. The rabbi makes a few factual errors in his eulogy but seems fairly sincere for someone who had never met the deceased. He says we aren't supposed to do eulogies on the eve of the Sabbath, and proceeds to give one. Jewish indirection is the mother of passive-aggressive behavior.

And of course I run out of pills in Syracuse. I didn't bring any Ativan, a big mistake. I was planning on refilling my prescriptions on Friday. I always wait until the last possible moment. I have enough AZT for the weekend. I'm up to six Zovirax a day and I have only four to last me the weekend.

I used to have the best insurance in the world. It covered doctors' visits and medication at 100 percent, after a miserable $100 deductible, which I was usually able to fulfill by January 10. Now it's the standard 80–20 plan. Each prescription costs $7.50, which isn't much, but still it adds up, considering I have three standard ones each month, and the occasional penicillin substitute and alpha interferon, and I was getting intranasal peptide T for neuropathy from the PWA Health Group at $65 a month, but it didn't really do much, so I stopped.

My mother's first cousin comes over to visit the family the following day. He's had five heart attacks in the past three years. He's had bypass surgery. His doctor said he recovered well and should expect ten more good years. I nod with him. He thought three years at best. I realize that's what I think my life expectancy is. And he has grandchildren. It's chilling. I should have grandchildren. Then I remember I am a homosexual and it isn't in the cards anyway.

I am terrified that I may have to spend another night in Syracuse. On Sunday we have another mild snowstorm, and the airport is about to close. My flight is canceled because the plane was diverted to Buffalo. The following flight is canceled. Luckily I am able to slip on the previous plane, which has been stalled on the runway for two hours. My cousin takes a taxi back to my aunt's two hours later.

Memorials come in twos and threes. For a while we referred to the obituary pages as the "gay sports pages"; we would turn to them first, scanning names to see if we knew anyone. Once Michael Morrissey called me at ten, asking if I'd seen a death notice. "I missed it."

"Oh, I see you only read the celebrity obituaries."

Now, out of guilt, I diligently go through the paid announcements in *The New York Times*.

We would read between the lines to see whether AIDS was the unspoken cause of death: if the person died at an early age, if there were no survivors or longtime companions listed, if pneumonia or lymphoma or any one of several opportunistic infections was mentioned, and so on. Now, even though more often people are forthright enough to mention "complications from AIDS," there is a stunning lack of urgency surrounding this disease. Our lives are imploding into silence. The walking wounded are trapped behind glass.

I am angry because the deaths keep piling up.

I am angry at the government for the continuing travel and immigration exclusion of HIV-positive people, which led the government to house hundreds of Haitian political refugees in a concentration camp at Guantanamo Bay for over a year, until the courts ruled this imprisonment unconstitutional.

I am angry at drug companies like Hoffmann–La Roche that

sit on valuable treatments and charge exorbitant prices for others.

I am angry at Senator Jesse Helms, who has done so much damage by imposing his perverted sense of morality on this country and taken away funding for sexually explicit safer-sex information that could have saved countless lives.

I am angry at Cardinal O'Connor for interfering with safer-sex education in the New York school system and promoting bigotry by denouncing the Rainbow curriculum.

But most of all I am angry because Bob Rafksy's prediction came true. He never spoke at another memorial after Tom Cunningham's. Bob Rafsky, my hero, died on February 21, 1993.

••

I wrote this piece for Details *magazine. It was due on February 15; I handed in the first draft about a month later. For a while, I was considering writing it in the form of an apology: "Please excuse David for being late with this article as he has had some difficulties of late," signed by my mother. But, of course, this is yet another piece that I would rather my mother never read.*

If anything, my antipathy against organized religion has grown in the past few years. The only time I find myself in church is for a memorial service. Bob Rafsky's memorial was held in the Quaker Friends Meeting House in Gramercy Park. It was highlighted by a disruption that should place it in the Hall of Fame of Memorials from Hell. After a video was shown documenting his AIDS activism and his relationship with his family, especially with his daughter, Bob's last boyfriend took to the lectern and claimed that Bob's love for his ex-wife was a "fake love." The boyfriend felt that he had been overlooked by the family in the aftermath of Bob's death, although they had broken up months earlier. He felt that the video had glossed over Bob's gay identity. Bob's ex-wife had just finished speaking; his parents were sitting in the front row. Everyone was totally appalled, but the etiquette of memorial services dictates that no one interrupt or dispute any reminiscence. For Bob

Rafsky, however, I think it would have been appropriate to disrupt his old boyfriend.

Jim Lewis also died as I was writing this piece. I was unable to incorporate his death into this piece: To include it would defuse the importance of Bob Rafsky's death. That's the problem with this endless epidemic: It is impossible to give each individual death the attention it deserves. Jim was the editor of The Body Positive magazine and co-author of the seminal piece "You Are Not Alone" that appears in every issue. I found I was unable to speak at his memorial. I think the only time I can actually have the presence of mind to say something about a dead friend is during an ACT UP death announcement. The Monday after a member of ACT UP dies, we have on-the-spot mini-memorials during our meetings, when people from the floor stand and provide personal reminiscences. These are always contained, confined within the three-and-a-half hour agenda of the meetings; they generally last no longer than fifteen minutes. We end these memorials by chanting "ACT UP, fight back, fight AIDS!" three times.

Response to the article was very favorable. One friend had a minor objection about my saying that Binky came with a fifty-year warrantee. His sister had been killed by a drunk driver ten years ago. Nonetheless, I told him it was probable that he would outlive me. We agreed that the survivor would donate five dollars to a charity he found personally loathsome that the deceased favored.

Shortly after my article came out, Harold "The Oldest Living Confederate with AIDS" Brodkey told all to The New Yorker in a second annual installment. The government pays farmers not to grow certain crops; I wonder whether the NEA would consider giving Harold Brodkey a grant to stop writing about AIDS.

My longtime relationship with my doctor ended abruptly in December 1993. He called me to tell me my crypto titers had risen.

"Cryptosporidiosis?" I inquired.

"No, cryptococcal meningitis."

He put me on Diflucan as prophylaxis. I, of course, began experiencing imaginary fevers and headaches that evening. I was to see him two weeks later to check on my blood. His office manager called the day before. My *doctor had to cancel due to a "medical emergency." I subsequently found out that he was in the hospital. He closed his practice. He died in January. My new doctor practices in the Village. His offices are next door to the rooming house where my first boyfriend lived—ironically, the most probable site of my original HIV infection.*

Michael Morrissey died on April 14, 1994. I found out he had died by reading the paid announcements in The New York Times. *He held fabulous parties every February. The invitation to his final party had a photo of him walking in a cobblestone alley in Italy. He wrote at the bottom of the photo: "I'm going to that corner and turn. Promise not to watch me go beyond that corner."*

David P.

I promised David P. I would tell his story. But how can you summarize a life in a few paragraphs? How can you attempt to encapsulate an individual's essence in a few brief pages? Any attempt will necessarily fall short. I want to write more than a mere memoir of disintegration, the irreversible decline of David P. I want to capture some part of David in print. I fear I am destined to fail. The best I can do is try to create a few snapshots from a history all too brief.

I am writing this to pay tribute to a friend. I am writing this because I miss David P. I am writing this because I am compelled to write it.

In these horrible times we have been forced to abbreviate the mourning process. How many people can you grieve for properly when everyone is dying? I wrote a novel for Jim Bronson, whom I barely knew. I wrote stories about my friends Saul Meissler, Glenn Peter Pumilia, and Glenn Person. Now I am reduced to brief essays in memoriam. Eventually all will be reduced to nothing but a litany of names chanted at the Quilt, panels of cloth the size of a coffin.

• • •

I was David B. and he was David P. We met at work. He was in typesetting; I was in the computer department. There was always something special about David P. He was the warmest person I knew. David P. was warm oatmeal, fresh bread, and home-made lemonade all in one, with a soft furry cat purring in your lap. I craved him like a drug.

David grew up in Connecticut. In the late seventies, he lived a block away from the Ramrod in the Village. I used to tease him about his scandalous life. "We were all wild and crazy then," he told me, half-kidding, half-serious. I would tell him my own shocking stories of depravity. He would chide me jokingly, "Congratulations. You've done it again. Five minutes with you, and we're back in the gutter."

I gave him a scandalous calendar for his thirtieth birthday. Expecting the party to be composed strictly of gay males, I came armed with some fag version of a *Sports Illustrated* swimsuit calendar. His lover, Wayne, catered. There was a wonderful mix of people, men and women, including his sister Susan. Embarrassed, I sneaked out before he opened my gift. Next week at work he told me the calendar was a hit. Everyone watched as he paged through it, month by month.

David had bizarre gastrointestinal problems for years before he was diagnosed with AIDS. He was in and out of work for quite some time, as doctors ran exhaustive and inconclusive tests to determine what the problem was.

I don't know how he was able to handle it when Wayne got sick. They were two heroes, caring for each other in the face of inhuman adversity. Is it worse to die or to survive your lover's death, knowing you will go through the same hell he went through?

Wayne didn't have many friends. Four of us from work drove upstate to the funeral. The service was in a beautiful rustic church. Wayne's mother lived nearby. At the cemetery, David stood silently behind dark sunglasses. Susan helped him back to the car afterward, as if David were a movie star ready to collapse at any moment.

Eventually he had to quit his job.

David stayed on, working part-time, just long enough to cover the insurance payments and stay on disability. We would meet for dinner at the Little Mushroom Cafe in Sheridan Square. David told me about the knitting group he was in, organized by GMHC. Six men would be quietly knitting in a room. Then simultaneously, six pillbox alarms would go off. Everyone popped his AZT tabs, then resumed knitting.

Through the months the group got smaller and smaller. Meetings were skipped when the instructor had to go to the hospital. Eventually they stopped meeting when they had dwindled down to two. The instructor died shortly thereafter.

David would visit his parents in Florida. It wasn't pleasant. His father, an alcoholic, would pretend that nothing was wrong. His mother would weep.

I took a long lunch and went up to Lenox Hill Hospital to see David. David had pneumonia again. Jim Bronson had died there three years earlier. Kathy, the personnel director at work, couldn't see him. She had problems with hospitals. She had masses said for him.

Terry from work was visiting David and they both saw a former employee sauntering up the street one evening at around six o'clock. David planned on inviting me at the same time the following evening so I would see her, too. We didn't get along. I was terrified at the prospect of ever seeing her again. Luckily we didn't cross paths.

David moved to Montclair, New Jersey, that fall. I took a bus from Port Authority one Saturday afternoon to see him. I was paranoid

I would miss the stop and be lost in New Jersey. One of his kitties hid in the closet. I recognized the poster of different species of fungi in the kitchen from his apartment in Brooklyn. We went out to the movies and then went for a drive through the neighborhood.

David was supposed to die three years ago. He was visiting his sister in Philadelphia when he fell ill with an infection. The personnel manager and her boss took a train to the hospital one afternoon to say good-bye. Miraculously, he recovered. When Brian at work heard David was dying, he said with resignation, "He's been sick for so long. Perhaps it's just as well. He's suffered long enough."

I wanted to slug Brian. "You fucking coldhearted gay Republican. Damn you!" I muttered to myself. "Don't be so cavalier with someone else's life. I bet you feel you're doing the right thing with your life. Sure, you occasionally send a check to GMHC. You buy a ribbon once a year for the PWA Coalition. You attend the Gay Pride parade if it isn't your weekend at the beach. You worry that the straights will get the wrong impression from drag queens. Damn you, you stupid selfish pig. Damn you to hell!"

I've never forgiven him for this.

David's neuropathy grew worse. He couldn't continue living alone. He moved in with Susan and her husband in a suburb of Boston. I saw him more often in Boston than when he lived in New Jersey. We drove out to Boston the weekend before the New Hampshire primary for an ACT UP demo. My friend Wayne dropped me off at Harvard Square and I took a bus to David's house. He and I sat in the living room and talked the usual trash. He couldn't button his clothes without assistance. He liked his home-infusion specialist. He could grip a glass only with the assistance of a thick polystyrene container.

David was on foscarnet for years. He was one of the first patients on the experimental protocol. Foscarnet was to stave off CMV and is so delivered intravenously through a Hickman catheter in the chest. Each drip took several hours. David had a few infections at the catheter site. David was already practically blind in one eye. His arms and legs were as skinny as twigs.

David loved his kitties. They gave him strength when his lover, Wayne, died and he moved to Montclair, New Jersey. They nourished his soul when he moved in with his sister in Cambridge. Perhaps the hardest thing of all was leaving them when he decided eventually to move to a hospice in Boston.

Each step he made was difficult: quitting his job, moving to Montclair, moving in with his sister in Cambridge, and now moving to the hospice. Susan was going back to school and her husband was teaching in another state. Suppose he fell down during the day and couldn't get up?

He found a boyfriend the last year of his life. His buddy from Boston's AIDS Action Council fell in love with him. It was a gift for both of them. They both thought carefully and seriously about a relationship. It was inadvisable from the point of view of AAC. Clients are not supposed to get involved with their buddies. There should be a distance to prevent the unbearable pain of loss. But how could they deny themselves this pleasure?

And so it was that much more difficult for David to enter the hospice. He felt he was letting Mike down. He told me that if not for Mike, he would have gone more easily.

A few months later I went to Boston under some pretext. It was really just to see David. I got my friend Neal to drive me to the hospice. It was a nice facility. But people were dying all the time. That was the worst, David P. told me. It's so depressing.

He always brightened up when I saw him.

• • •

I was a pallbearer at his funeral. Never wear long shoelaces if you are to be a pallbearer. You will trip. His lover, Mike, sat in the front row at the memorial service. I ran into Mike a few months later, at a bar in Cambridge. He was doing fine. He missed David P. a lot.

After David died, Mary the office manager said, "Promise me you won't get sick. I don't think I can go through this again."

Mary was everyone's second mother.

How can you say this to me? I've gone through this so many times I've lost count. Of course I'm going to get sick. Don't be absurd. But Mary is the mother we've never had. With mixed emotions, I lied. "I promise."

On
the
Drip

My regular doctor is in Palm Springs, Wyoming, or at some international conference. I see his charming solicitous partner whose overly concerned demeanor sometimes gives me the creeps. Reading my chart, he recommends that I should consider IVGG: intravenous gamma globulin. Gamma globulin is a protein active against cancer and viral and bacterial infections. It's another part of the immune system, along with T-4 cells. I would make an excellent candidate for this protocol: I have fewer than 100 T-cells and have a history of susceptibility to bacterial infections. His patients on gamma globulin have all managed to stave off CMV infections. I don't particularly feel like getting strep or Hemophilus again, especially after that penicillin nightmare in January 1993.

I tell him I'll think about it.

I think about it.

I am completely terrified.

But if it keeps me off a catheter and daily infusions of ganciclovir or foscarnet, fine.

According to Paul Monette, ganciclovir is now commonly delivered with a pump, not a hanging IV. First toothpaste got the pump, then sneakers got the pump; now it's used for CMV prophylaxis.

I don't mind needle pricks, but an infusion is another matter. I've always had good veins. Back in college, I used to donate large quantities of blood for purposes other than clinical tests. The nurses would always compliment my veins. It's no big deal for me to give two, three, or four test tubes of blood every time I see my doctor. Once my friend Chris, terrified, got me to go with him to the clinic for some complicated protocol. I took the afternoon off from work and waited with him in one of those molded-plastic chairs used in health clinics, fast-food restaurants, and waiting rooms for visiting incarcerated felons in medium-security facilities. Eventually, Chris was called. I joined him as he underwent the procedure. The physician stuck a needle into Chris's arm and took some blood. Big deal.

I decide to wait until I see my regular doctor again.

A month later, my doctor concurs. He also recommends pentamidine infusions, twice monthly. The best prophylaxis against PCP is Bactrim, available in tablets; unfortunately, I'm allergic. I don't feel like going through the desensitization procedure that my doctor suspects won't work on me anyway. I've been inhaling pentamidine for a few years. I tried it at home for a few months, but didn't feel comfortable with it. I would constantly put off doing my inhalation: I would always be a week or ten days late. It didn't feel right. I didn't get that same bitter taste in the back of my throat.

I tell him I'll think about it.

I ask my friend Wayne, the relentless top and control queen who giggles incessantly. Wayne works for the PWA Health Group, which sold me those underground ddC pills that ended up being variably dosed. He says it might be a good thing. The Health Group is selling Kemron (a formulation of oral alpha interferon developed in Kenya); although it is almost assuredly ineffective, it is Wayne's duty in his capacity of guaranteeing quality control that their Kemron be a placebo of proper strength and chemical derivation.

A billion years ago I recall protesting with ACT UP against the pediatric protocol for intravenous immunoglobulin. Infants were getting four-hour drips of IVIG once a month to see if this would help their immune systems against bacterial infections. However, to be scientifically objective, some scientist had decided that in order to avoid the placebo effect, where, given any drug whether useful or not, the patient feels psychologically better, half of the infants received a four-hour sugar drip once a month, putting them at risk of infection from the IV. This was barbaric.

Eventually IVIG was approved for infants and children.

Insurance companies balk at paying for gamma globulin because it's so expensive and it's currently approved only for children. The home-care nurse will be around $400; and the actual substance is around $1,500. There are other infusions for which a nurse can drop off the equipment, set you up, then go to a diner or a matinee performance of the latest Bruce Willis disaster and then return to unhook you. Pentamidine and gamma globulin are the only two infusions that require the presence of a nurse for the duration of the infusion, to monitor for possible allergic reactions.

Gamma globulin is the same thing as immunoglobulin.

Those poor kids suffered so I could try this. I feel guilty. I'm just another overprivileged gay white male with a cushy job and private insurance. Suspicious of the high prices, and slightly taken aback by my doctor's enthusiasm, I wonder if kickbacks are part of the deal. Is this another insurance scam? I don't know anyone else on this protocol. I have a feeling you couldn't get gamma globulin on Medicare. But it's not as if everybody can gain access to d4T, which is still in phase-three trials. Am I just wallowing in Jewish-liberal guilt combined with survival guilt? Should I continue to wallow in it? Better to wallow alive than dead.

Before my first infusion, I have to undergo a nutritional counseling session at Hemasuction's office. I schedule it for 1:00 P.M., during my lunch hour. What could be more appropriate? I had been planning on seeing a nutritionist for the past three years, but I never got around to it. I was a little leery of the ones my friends recommended, especially the vegetarians on kelp diets. Well, one less item to check off from my "to do" list.

I generally try to schedule appointments during lunch or right after work. I seem to have so many appointments with so many doctors that I fear I'll use up all my sick time on regularly scheduled checkups. I also like to keep a little flexibility for those ubiquitous demos I just can't stop myself from going to. And it would be nice to have an occasional vacation. I'm saving those days off from work for a rainy day, and I fear the extended weather forecast is ominous. If I hadn't moved from that hellhole in Hell's Kitchenette and done the yuppie co-op thing, I wouldn't have to worry about time off at all: I'd probably be on disability. Edmund White himself, the reigning queen of gay literature, according to *Time* magazine, where he mysteriously grew to six feet (I'm sure I was mistaken, due to his bad posture), even asked me why I was still working and not just writing before some benefit where we were reading a few months ago. I don't know. Fear of poverty, I guess. Maybe an element of mortal terror of the standard health care in the U.S. for the underprivileged.

I can schedule infusions at home, after work. That means three fewer days a month at the gym. Not that I'm compulsive or anything. The gym thing has sort of gone to hell this past year. Three times a week is a reasonable goal now.

As usual, I bring my anal-retentive self to the Hemasuction office five minutes early. There's no way to go cross-town with public transportation. I have to rush through the jackhammer-filled streets of Manhattan on a balmy afternoon.

It's April 21, Secretaries' Day, which means the entire support staff is out for lunch indefinitely. My nutritional counselor ushers me into her office at twenty minutes past one. I'd be fine if I had eaten something since nine-thirty, because I'm slightly hypoglycemic. My friend Glenn Person always carried an apple in his backpack. But then, he was a triathlete who burned up to 4,000 calories a day. He died of AIDS back in 1987, half a year after completing the Ironman in Hawaii.

Nancy L. (R.N., M.S.) hands me an easy-to-read booklet about nutrition for people with HIV. It's written in basic English. No Proustian memoirs here. Patiently, she goes over the information in the booklet, a health teacher giving a watered-down lecture with slides for the benefit of the slower members of the class. Surely she's not addressing her concerns toward me? I'll listen out of politeness. She seems to be talking to someone who's already on death's doorstep. I look around and realize it's a class of one.

Am I deluding myself? Am I really sick? Is this stage fifteen of denial? Should I continue the ruse of working and working out? Why waste these last few remaining years, days, hours, in a heinous job, when I could be devoting all my time to writing? Perhaps because I seem to write only about AIDS, and that would make it that much worse, more present.

I lie about my general eating habits. Well, I stretch the truth. I pretend I have been following the American Association of Dietary Fiber and General Roughage's Minimum Adult Daily Requirements religiously. I always eat a well-balanced combination from the seven food groups. I don't eat more than two eggs a week. I have pork only on alternate Tuesdays. I go crazy for big, leafy vegetables. I chew on birch bark to aid digestion thrice daily. But I throw in some snacks just so it will sound plausible. An oatmeal cookie at four. A brownie before bed. And Nancy likes this, even more than my hypothetical well-balanced meals.

Instead of orange juice for breakfast, she suggests one of those nectars loaded with calories. Eat at McDonald's, she continues. Eat your favorite foods. Maybe put on five or ten extra pounds. It's always better to have that margin of safety.

Make foods more caloric. Try Carnation Instant Breakfast. Add milk powder to beverages. Carry around a few granola bars. Use blue cheese or Russian dressing.

To my chagrin, I find that not only is sushi outlawed (I knew that: deadly toxo lurks in raw fish), but so is brie. Soft, runny cheeses are on the list of no-nos. Hysterical, that afternoon I call up my very best friend in the whole world, John Palmer Weir, Jr. "How can I be a card-carrying homo without brie?"

"There's still quiche," he points out. "We'll always have quiche."

"Thank God," I say. "I thought it was Paris," I mutter to myself.

"Check your weight once a week. Watch out for wasting syndrome," warns Nancy. Sure. I'll do my best to keep on the lookout. And I promise never again to get anxious or think of the word *elephant*.

Gamma globulin can take up to four hours; pentamidine can take up to two. I schedule my first two infusions for 5:30 P.M. on successive days one week after my nutritional counseling, which means I have to leave for work at precisely 8:30 A.M. because it takes exactly thirty minutes to walk to work, including a stop to pick up breakfast (poppy-seed bagel with butter, orange juice) and the newspapers *(The New York Times, New York Newsday)*. I'm a little nervous. Binky will be there. He was on his way to Florida for a four-day vacation when he remembered that tomorrow was Davey's first infusion and he decided to come back. I could have asked him, but asking is so difficult for me, because I have heard the word *no* too many times, for the silliest of favors. I asked him if he could take the day off when we moved, and he didn't see why it was that important. "What do you need me for? We have movers." Well, he was in a bad mood because he had to teach a masters' class the day before the April 25 March on Washington and couldn't fly to D.C. because everything was booked and he didn't enjoy crowds in any event. So that Sunday he took off to Florida to visit some friends, who hadn't returned his phone calls because they were still in D.C. I returned from D.C. to see a note on the table. Binky said he would be away for four days. I mentally adjusted my schedule. When the boyfriend's away, the mice will play. I started planning a toga party for Tuesday, and a pool party in the Jacuzzi for Wednesday. Then I remembered I had infusions scheduled on both those nights. He called later that night and told me he was coming back on Monday.

Our latest knock-down drag-out concerned our housewarming. I know we should have discussed it before Binky was faced with the absurd image of my alphabetizing the ninety-five invitations on the floor. I invited everyone that I've fantasized not exchanging bodily fluids with in the past five years, and a few women, too. Binky wanted to invite only those he would feel comfortable donating ten pints of blood to if they were in a car wreck. We should have had separate parties: one for those who reside in Chelsea, another for ACT UP members, another for pseudonymous drag columnists (both were on Fire Island that Sunday, of course), another one for writers, and another one for HIV-positives.

Nurse Perry calls me at work, apologizing. He doesn't want to disturb me on the job, but he's running late today.

Perry comes rolling a steel IV holder down the hallway at ten minutes to six, with boxes and boxes of gifts and exciting new houseware products. Only this time it isn't Hanover House, UPS, or International Male: It's Hemasuction. It's my lucky day! Seventy-five booklets filled with S&H green stamps, and I'm getting my own IV. Should I name it Iman or Twiggy?

"This is yours to keep." I'm so excited. "We try to respect your privacy. The neighbors, and all. We'll only be wheeling it in once. Some people use a nail in the ceiling instead of the IV pole." I figure that might cause a crimp in terms of mobility.

"Is it sturdy enough for a sling? I'm sorry, I guess I need two. Binky, would you mind signing up? You'll get your free IV pole, too, and then we can experiment." It's too tall for the bathroom shelves. I have to stick it in the dark, deep recesses of the closet in the bedroom. Can one hang a chandelier from it? I guess it will be useful for Maypole dances and tetherball games.

My visceral reaction is the same a property owner would have after finding out that the city was planning on opening an out-patient methadone clinic next door. NIMBY: Not in My Backyard. I never wanted to have a PC in my apartment; they remind me too much of my loathsome nine-to-five job, which involves data-processing equipment. But after my boss was fired I bought one, assuming that I was next in line, or that I would valiantly quit in protest of his firing. That was more than five years ago. Now my apartment is suffused with pills, prescriptions, pharmaceuticals, and prophylactic devices, medical and otherwise. The mirrored bathroom cabinet is nearly bursting with salves, ointments, and drugs. It's a good thing that Binky isn't a hypochondriac. Mercifully, he has escaped the homosexual addiction to expensive skin- and hair-care products that so many are afflicted with. There just isn't any room. If he were HIV-positive, perhaps we could share prescriptions as well as tank tops.

Perry gives me an allergy kit filled with decongestants, anti-inflammatories, hydrocortisones, and steroids. The supplies come in a box with the Hemasuction insignia. Unfortunately for me, the insignia is on the top and the bottom of the box, so when I flatten it out for recycling, it shows no matter on which side I turn it. Instead of putting it in the compacter room on my floor, I stash it downstairs after midnight with the rest of the recyclables. Thank God for my housewares-supply shelves. I rhapsodize once more on the miles of tiles and endless storage space that Leonard, the former owner of this apartment, has bequeathed me. The infectious-waste container will be stored on the floor of the supply closet, in the back.

"Now, which one of you is David?" asks Perry.

"He is," we say, pointing at each other.

Perry and Binky manage to pry me from the ceiling a good twenty minutes later. I leave claw marks in the paint.

Perry has a British accent. He may or may not be a repressed or closeted homosexual. He's a bit stuffy; he seems to have mild vestiges of that class thing going on: the neighborhood deteriorating, the slightly stiff and superior poise, and all. But I feel no prick when he sticks me.

I look away as he sticks me. I don't like the sight of blood, especially my own. I used to stare as my doctor took my blood, and watch it fill the tubes. "It's quite warm, people don't expect that," he said as he handed me several tubes to drop off with the receptionist. I imagine it's the image of an icy-cold test tube. Blood comes out bright crimson and then bleeds to wine-dark red. I avert my eyes. They remain averted for a long time. Finally, Binky can't resist telling me in a sarcastic voice, "You can look now."

Perry comes to the rescue. "You're next."

I want to be in the ads in *The New England Journal of Medicine* for trouble-free infusion: riding a horse, swimming, at the discotheque, even having my period. I want to be photographed by Annie Leibovitz dragging an IV pole with fluids behind me as I water-ski in the latest Gap wear. I live for publicity. But at the last moment I lose my nerve and tell Binky I'd rather he not take a photo for the album delineating my decline and fall: Davey's First Infusion, smiling ever so bravely, fighting against tears, one arm held high in mock strength: For those of us who are about to infuse, we salute you.

During the infusion there are questions to answer, there is paperwork to sign. Perry is my personal flight attendant, armed with a mélange of items and busywork to keep me amused during the flight. I wait in vain for a first-class upgrade to a pump infusion, or at least for my complimentary soft drink and foil-wrapped peanuts.

I have one pathetic moment: dragging the IV behind me as I go to the bathroom. In that moment I feel like all my friends who've ever been in the hospital. Many never got out. I feel like my grandmother in the Jewish Home for the Aged.

I am left with a bruise on my right arm on the inside of my el-
bow. I'll just say that my boyfriend and I are exploring our sexuality in new directions that involve electrical cables and bludgeons.
I consider marking the sites of future infusions in a connect-the-
dots motif so after six months I will have a serviceable tattoo or at
least a minor constellation.

Perry warns me that I may be peeing a lot with all this extra fluid.
I wake up the next morning with an erection, which, alas, dissipates after I urinate. I used to wake up almost always with an
erection (preferably not my own). This hardly ever happens now.
    Some people report a huge boost of energy after gamma glob-
ulin. With me, it is less a burst of energy than a lack of utter exhaustion. For the past few months I would drag myself home after
work and desperately need to lie down for a half hour. I feel more
as if I've stabilized to something close to normal—perhaps what
I've been missing the past two years without even realizing it.
Okay, so I scrubbed the tiles in the bathroom for five hours—is
that unusual? Perhaps for me, who finds a scrub brush as alien as
a clitoris. I have been exclusively homosexual for the past thirty-
six years, and am not about to break a perfect record.

The following night I get my first pentamidine infusion. It is over
in an hour. Everything tastes a bit rank and metallic after the pentamidine, for a day or so.

I stuff my gym clothes and towel into the plastic bag with the
Hemasuction logo and force myself to take it to the gym. I want
to accept this next stage as soon as possible.

"Be prepared" is my motto. Which is why I rushed home after
work—I didn't want to miss my infusion—and stacked the six
new CDs on my CD player, including the new super-air-brushed
Lulu, which looks as if she uses Wite-Out instead of makeup,

made sure I had enough reading material and letters to answer, and then I sank into the futon couch, and of course I could not leave without assistance. Wayne came over in the middle of the infusion with the wrong brand of ginger ale and mandarin-orange flavored seltzer water. (Is it possible to be allergic to mandarin-orange flavor?) At least he didn't get peach. So we sat and giggled and looked at photographs in my album, and I apologized for not walking him to the door, since I was encumbered, and he left, and then of course he came back five minutes later because he forgot his sunglasses, which were right on the table, and I had to drag my fucking IV to the door, and it got caught and twisted, and I made faces like the eleven-year-old girl in the movie *Airplane* whose IV keeps getting dislodged when the singing nun strums her guitar and swings it for the entertainment of the plane. I love Wayne. I guess he should have my keys. Binky gets angry whenever I give keys away. I guess that's because that's how we got together. I gave him my keys too early.

My very best friend in the entire world, John Palmer Weir, Jr., to whom my entire writing output is dedicated, came over to sit through the second pentamidine, which was a total of only forty-five minutes of drip. I always used to watch the needles; now I just avert my eyes. But John Weir was making a conscious effort to show me that nothing human offended him; he wanted to show me it was okay. I knew it was okay. I asked him, but *noooooooo*, he had to stare in shock and horror and revulsion as Manny the nurse stuck me, and Manny wasn't that used to doing this sort of thing in the home environment because even though I have excellent veins—indeed, I've entered them in competitions and always gotten at least honorable mention—he was used to hospitals, Perry said, where the patient can be tied down with straps or something or other, and he stabbed me and I bled and John's eyes turned to saucers, and even though I didn't want to look it was as if his eyes were reflecting what was going on, which I didn't want to know; one could see the depth of the sorrow and the pity; it was like watching a twenty-hour movie about the Holocaust in his eyes. Manny tells me that he had a wonderful time skiing in Colorado last winter, and I stifle the impulse to tell him how politically incorrect it is of him to travel to Colorado: Hasn't he heard of the boycott? What about the political ramifications? Because he is the one sticking the needle into me.

Afterward John Weir admitted it wasn't particularly pleasant watching me get sticked. I chided him repeatedly, which both of us enjoyed, as we are unnatural. But afterward we went and saw the new Sharon Stone movie, which was really the new William Baldwin movie, in which he relinquished his shirt repeatedly and he was so entrancing we have no idea at all how badly he acted.

Next month I plan on watching the entire Galsworthy saga on videocassette. Unfortunately, I've run out of William Baldwin movies.

And now I can't stop eating. I never miss my cookie snack in the afternoon, my brownie before bedtime. I'm gaining weight at an appallingly slow rate. Farewell, flat stomach, forever. I fear it would bode ill should it ever reappear, for that would mean I was back on the way down, approaching my Christ-on-the-Cross-in-Auschwitz phase. More likely I will end up with a bloated Biafran belly. Too much gas.

My hunger is uncontrollable. Like Marilyn Chambers, I'm insatiable. I am eating when I'm not even hungry. I have subconsciously internalized the *Diseased Pariah News* maxim "Get fat, don't die!" Like Sylvia Plath, I eat men like air. My sexual hunger has been displaced. And when I become too weak to cook and shop and the boyfriend is anywhere but here, I can always thank heaven for takeout.

But somewhere in the pit of my stomach, I worry. Will my fragile physical equilibrium allow this to happen? I don't think so.

• • •

I can think of few sights more terrifying than my itemized statement from Chubb dated 6-15-93, covering three infusions. The bill totaled $3,923.35. Five items listed under medical supplies totaling $3,503.35 are marked with code 53: "Pending receipt of information requested from other sources." The remaining item, "Registered nurse," is marked code 13: "Benefits are limited to the reasonable and customary amount." Chubb feels that $75 is reasonable for a registered nurse, not $300; $75 covered at 80 percent yields $60. Thus Chubb is issuing a draft to Apple Stat for $60 out of a bill for $3,923.35.

After seventeen frantic phone calls to Hemasuction, Chubb LifeAmerica, my doctor, my accountant, my crisis-intervention counselor, my personal trainer, and the Psychic HelpLine, the situation is straightened out. As the Clintons hold a series of private meetings to determine how this country will achieve universal health care, I sit on my futon couch and stare at the plastic bag of precious liquid as it drips into my arm; I sit huddled into a tiny ball, still as a statue, emotionally distraught, wondering who the hell is going to pay for my next infusion.

The
AIDS Clone
vs. the
New Clone

A fad is ten minutes, a trend is six months, but a clone is forever. Clones have been with us since Stonewall, the dawn of Modern Gay Time. Throughout the seventies we saw the rise of the circuit queen (henceforth referred to as Clone Classic) with his mirrored sunglasses, tight jeans, gym body, and severe haircut. The Clone Classic was found in gyms, discos, and on Fire Island. One of the three memorable *Christopher Street* cartoons captured this phenomenon with a drawing of six clones captioned: "Why gay men are seldom identified in police lineups." The late eighties gave us the New Clone, with his multiple earrings, backward baseball cap, gym body, and severe haircut. The New Clone could be found at the gym, at ACT UP meetings, at Queer Nation demonstrations, and on Fire Island. In the postmodern nineties perhaps fifty percent of the gay men in New York City are seropositive. Inevitably, health status has mutated into a fashion statement. Witness the comparisons.

Originally appeared in Diseased Pariah News, *Issue 9, Winter 1993/4.*

The New Clone

Last vacation: two weeks in Provincetown

Inhales nitrous oxide

Antioxidant: Clinique skin cream

Blender drink: margaritas

Takes recreational drugs

Fashion choice: Galanos gowns

Most recent semi-permanent body disfigurement that required sedation: nipple piercing

Leisure activity: attending media press conferences

Angry because couldn't get into Mr. Fuji's Tropicana

Last book read: *Last Exit to Brooklyn*

Spasmodic motion at 3:00 A.M.: dancing, Sound Factory Bar

Easily bored

Wears loose-fit Levi's Silver Tab jeans

The AIDS Clone

Last vacation: two weeks at Lenox Hill

Inhales aerosol pentamidine

Antifungals: Lotrisone, clotrimazole

Blender drink: ddI and orange juice

Takes prescription drugs

Fashion necessity: hospital gowns

Most recent semi-permanent body disfigurement that required sedation: Hickman catheter implant

Leisure activity: attending medical forums

Angry because couldn't get into gp160 protocol

Last book read: *Final Exit*

Spasmodic motion at 3:00 A.M.: epileptic seizure

Tires easily

Wears baggy clothes

The New Clone

Changing the sheets at 4:00 A.M. after hot sex with a guy he picked up at the Bijou

Favorite movie: *Blade Runner*, director's cut

Least-favorite homo in history: Roy Cohn

Bald as a fashion statement

Pale skin: avoids the sun

Likes oral sex

Exercises at Better Bodies

Bitter because youth passed by

Doesn't speak to his family

Weight-loss secret: skipping dessert

Ex doesn't call because of bad attitude

The AIDS Clone

Changing the sheets at 4:00 A.M. after night sweats

Favorite movie: *Death Becomes Her*

Least-favorite homo in history: Roy Cohn

Bald from radiation therapy

Pale skin: anemic

Likes oral sex

Physical therapy at St. Luke's

Bitter because will bypass age

Doesn't speak to his family

Weight-loss secret: forgetting nutritional supplement

Ex doesn't call because he's dead

Wide
Sargasso
Sea

I don't know about you, but I appreciate hindsight. Not that I would ever sit on the throne of justice in all pomp and circumstance, dressed by the same couturier who clothes Queen Elizabeth, or perhaps Quentin Crisp, and dispense well-reasoned opinions about personal relationships and traumas after the fact, generally concluding with that tiresome, yet admittedly satisfying, adage, "I told you so." Revenge may be sweet, but a well-placed snide comment is true vindication.

But then I return to my natural state of guilt. Who am I to judge? How can I achieve personal growth with such a spiteful demeanor? Do I care? Perversely, I prefer the solipsistic approach of self-directed retrovision. After I screw up, as I invariably do, I like to repeat to myself, "I told myself so." I have only myself to blame.

If only I hadn't eaten fried rice for dinner after going ballistic at lunch and gorging myself at the salad bar; if only I hadn't asked the dental hygienist for a mint-flavored topical anesthetic while I was taking Flagyl for my latest gastrointestinal disorder; if only I hadn't eaten that last piece of chocolate—I might not be sitting on the cold, cold tile floor of the bathroom at eleven o'clock waiting for that next inevitable wave of disgust to leap from the throat into the porcelain goddess I lay myself prostate in worshipful attendance of, while Binky and his two sisters are applauding the final curtain of the Thursday-evening performance of *Jelly's Last Jam*.

In January I itched. In March I coughed. And in May I shat.

In January I itched for a week, a delayed hypersensitive reaction to a form of penicillin to which I was previously unallergic. My body was transformed into an ambulatory rash approximately sixty-eight inches tall, against which a battery of antihistamines and steroids proved ineffective.

In March I coughed through the night, due to some annoying postnasal drip rivaling the primordial ooze in both consistency and ubiquity, to the point of waking myself up at four in the morning in fits of hacking.

And in May I shat in a continuous stream, for what seemed like forever, but was probably not more than a week.

It began on Friday night. Should I attribute it to the individual-size cheesecake I got from the gourmet deli near work for dessert at lunch? I doubt the case that contained it was refrigerated. Or was it perhaps the twentieth nacho chip I had after work, visiting my friend Wayne at his office? I was still in that binge mode. I mean, I couldn't stop eating for fear of losing weight. The lessons of Hemasuction and Karen Carpenter weighed heavily on my subconscious. But eating more wasn't necessarily the solution, because I found my stomach was becoming more and more particular. I was becoming, horror of horrors, that fifties cinematic cliché: the sensitive homosexual. I was allergic to several forms of penicillin, sulfa drugs, several nucleoside analogues, and probably bran. My diet was becoming more and more rigid: If I didn't have exactly the same thing every day at exactly the same time (a banana, a sip of juice, and a handful of pharmaceuticals before work; a bagel, toasted, with butter and a pint of orange juice for breakfast; a turkey and provolone sandwich on a roll with a pint of apple juice and a brownie for lunch; pasta and salad and a glass of seltzer for dinner; perhaps a scoop of ice cream and a few noncaloric slurps on Binky's penis as a bedtime snack), all havoc might break loose.

Certain rules had to be followed. Peanut butter was a dangerous thing. Salad bars were to be avoided at all costs. Bran was completely out of the question. Too much candy led to certain evacuation. I am a designated beanless area. There is only so much chocolate a body can take.

My weight remained steady, my body-fat percentage constant.

And if I had too much of some forbidden fruit, my body, demonstrating a strict homeostasis, would rectify the situation immediately, with a brief outburst. Garbage in, garbage out. And a day or two later I would return to my normal state of sylphlike beauty.

But it was not normal, this diarrhea.

My stomach was bloated. Sure, my stomach has been distended for the past twelve years. I am a human flatulence machine. I always get the machine I want at the gym. Should I want privacy, I have found that a well-placed fart can clear the entire floor—although I admit I have had a few embarrassing moments in the hallway outside my office at work, due to involuntary voluble emissions.

Sometimes I feel my system has been unalterably changed after that night I drank a gallon of Colyte flavored with Crystal-Light lemonade in preparation for my M.D. Tusch–induced colonoscopy. For months excrement came out (as if my entire intestines were unrolled) in pieces large enough to cross the English Channel.

But this was different. I had diarrhea on Friday night at two-hour intervals. After an evening of stomach gurgling and typical premenstrual cramps, I made successive visits to the porcelain palace at 1:00 A.M., 3:00 A.M., 5:00 A.M., and 7:00 A.M. Thank God it was a weekend.

And these were liquid explosions.

This was not normal.

•   •   •

Sometimes it feels as if I'm seeing a doctor every week. Next week it's the dentist. I still have to make an appointment to see my ophthalmologist to make sure I haven't been victimized by CMV retinitis. The six-month reminder card is buried in my papers. And now with these infusions, that's three more blocks of time each month devoted to medical matters. At least I don't have to go to my doctor for pentam inhalation anymore. That's one less appointment.

I just saw my doctor on Wednesday. I asked about the possibility of transinterdigitoanal verrucae. I may have stuck my finger in someone's anus in the bathtub. Okay, okay, I know I should have worn finger cots, sterile surgical gloves, or at least Playtex Living rubber gloves. He replies, it's a different virus. You're more likely to transmit it to someone's penis by jerking him off. More good news for modern man. The doctor proceeds to inject an entire bottle of alpha interferon, twice what he has done before, directly into the warts on my hands. I stay home from work the following day with faux flu, a common side effect of the drug.

So of course I don't call my doctor for a few days. It just might go away.

Where did I get this bug? I wonder whether I have eaten brown foods. A big mistake. Shit can blend into the scenery. I wonder how I managed to avoid hepatitis last summer when everybody else seemed to get it. It's true, I have been a certified rim-free zone since January 23, 1982.

I have a confession to make.

I have never rimmed.

I may have lapped some Saran Wrap once or twice. But by the time I had conquered my cultural heritage of 5,762 years of Jewish prissiness, the moment of relatively carefree analingus had passed. Yes, I have been rimmed. And undoubtably I will spend another 10,000 years in Purgatory for not reciprocating.

Could I have been infected from the gamma globulin? Haven't

most of my ill effects been bad reactions to drugs up to this point? I remember back in the early eighties when people were blaming AIDS on the hepatitis B vaccine. When I finally call my doctor the following week, he admits that the alpha interferon could cause mild diarrhea for a day, but certainly not for the duration of my current affliction.

A week later I shriek "Are you clean?" at my boyfriend when he offers his metallic-tasting penis for my inspection, which I suspect he has been wrapping in aluminum foil until I realize that the Flagyl or maybe the pentamidine is altering my taste buds.

Dear Diary, Saturday was queasy. I swallowed my quota of Imodium tablets and feasted on toast and bottled water. On Friday at work I had promised my friend Tom I would help work on the sets of his new play. A promise is a promise. Armed with two tablets of Imodium, I stagger to the bus stop. I pick up a bottle of Canada Dry ginger ale. I do my requisite twenty-seven minutes of work (I have an alarmingly short attention span) and then I sit with Tom and watch a run-through of Act One. I seem okay. I pick up a muffin on the way home.

Sunday night is a repeat of Friday.

Monday I'm okay. Breakfast is a plain toasted bagel with bottled water; lunch is chicken soup. I clutch my stomach through the Monday-night ACT UP meeting, feel my complexion grow several shades paler. Why on earth do I force myself out on nights like these? Is the activist addiction that great?

Tuesday is bad-news day. I stay home from work. I'm rapidly using up my sick time. I call up my doctor. The possibility of being tested for amoebas looms its ugly head. I think I might as well get tested that very day. I wouldn't even have to take the horrifying amoeba-test laxative that I have written about in nauseatingly excruciating detail elsewhere.

I feel a little better on Wednesday. Staying home is so intensely boring, and there is nothing particularly engrossing on television. So on Wednesday I take the Perilous Journey to work.

I saw the Disney movie *The Perilous Journey* during my Wonder Bread years. A cat, a dog, and maybe a canary traveled thousands of miles to return home. My walk to work is a random walk, fraught with peril. At each intersection I either turn or go straight, depending on the traffic-light status, the intensity of the sun, the sound of street cleaners, car alarms, fire-truck sirens, and jackhammers, and the ambient presence of cute boys. I try to avoid Fourteenth Street. I almost always end up walking by Bed Bath & Beyond. GMHC's main office is all too frequently passed by. I don't want to be reminded on a daily basis of my future status of clienthood. If chance has me in front of Michael's Muffins on Seventh, I'll generally pick one up for breakfast; otherwise I'll steer myself toward Giant Bagels on University and Thirteenth.

But what was once a serendipitous perambulation has been transformed into the Perilous Journey. Will I make it to work, underwear intact? With each step, pressure builds up inside me and I have no idea whether it is shit or just air. Will I release noxious fumes to plosive sound, or will I soil myself with a slightly liquid fart?

It takes exactly thirty minutes to get to work, and there seems to be no way of ameliorating this situation. By bus it takes exactly thirty minutes, including the wait for the Broadway local at Twenty-third. By cab it takes exactly thirty minutes, given traffic conditions at rush hour. What do I do if the urge to evacuate strikes en route? It isn't so much an urge as a compulsion, an uncontrollable purgative.

There are no public toilets in New York City. Last year a company from France set up four experimental public toilets. Although they were a great success (clean, safe, and well stocked with toilet paper), unfortunately they were not wheelchair-accessible, and the City Council had to nix the idea of separate but equal toilets. I could plan a route leapfrogging from one coffee-house to another. Bars generally don't open until noon. The Community Center is closed, and the facilities are less than ideal.

The gym is a convenient pit stop: My membership card is worth its weight in gold.

A few words of practical advice:

1. Always carry a few Imodium pills in your backpack.
2. Toilet paper is always useful. Facial tissues are even better. Tucks are best.
3. That extra pair of underwear is crucial.

Dazed with hunger, I walk through Balducci's on the way home, looking at the assorted gourmet meals I can't eat, available at ten dollars a quarter-pound. Let's see: Will it be boiled rice and boiled chicken tonight? Or perhaps I should try the boiled-chicken-and-boiled-rice combination. There's always Campbell's chicken-and-rice soup, if only it didn't contain so much sodium and MSG. As an aperitif, I'm leaning toward bottled water, a domestic brand. Perrier is awfully tempting; unfortunately, it is a bit too effervescent for my present mood. Warm, flat ginger ale is always a treat. Unfortunately, the bottles in the supermarket are all properly sealed. I don't know if I could wait the requisite time for the ginger ale to air.

I am strangely constipated for the stool test on Thursday. I take only half the laxative. I assume that the mere sight of the noxious phosphate chemical would cause me to purge. But half is not enough. I read through *New York* magazine's twentieth-anniversary issue, cover to cover. No dice. I should have come on Tuesday, when a sip of bottled water would cause me to run to the john in moments, when an apple went through my system in twelve minutes flat.

After an hour and a half of senseless waiting and a futile walk around the block, I assume the classic enema position, which is not that different from the classic post-nuclear-holocaust duck-and-cover position. I lie curled up in the fetal position, staring at the gutter drain on the floor, clutching my legs, slowly squeezing the plastic bottle into an orifice rarely used for intake of any sort. It soon enough has the desired effect. The moment I return to my apartment, I explode.

On Friday I call my doctor to find out that results will not be complete until Monday. That leaves an entire weekend of uncertainty. I'm convinced it's cryptosporidiosis, and I will be hooked up to an IV in some hideous hospital while a hundred people come to the housewarming scheduled for Sunday.

I continue the bran diet: bananas, rice, apples, and toast.

There's that mad moment when I realize that my diet consists of nothing at all. Once the gastrointestinal tubes have been cleared, food slides through them as fast as a particle accelerator. Whatever I eat is gone in a minute. So I reduce myself to the jailhouse diet of bread and water. But my doctor tells me that preliminary tests have indicated I have yeast in my stool. I should avoid yeast. *Aaaaaaacccccchhhh!* A yeast infection! I realize I really am a lesbian. So scratch the bread. Just water. But my latest *Advocate* warns me against drinking tap water. There was an outbreak of cryptosporidiosis in Milwaukee last April. No treatment exists. Sixty-five percent of Milwaukee AIDS Project's seven hundred clients exhibited severe conditions connected with the cryptosporidiosis outbreak. Most vulnerable are HIV-infected people with T-4 cell counts of less than 100. That's me. I have all the major symptoms: watery, chronic, profuse diarrhea, often worsened by eating; dull, crampy upper abdominal pain, often worsened by eating. I am advised to act as if I'm in Mexico and brush my teeth with bottled water.

Yet even filtered water bottled in Poland Springs, Maine, produces a flood. Okay. I'll do the new diet: just air. And then I realize that even air isn't safe, what with airborne microbacteria that cause TB and MAI.

• • •

I find out that Dennis is coming to the housewarming with Julio, and his friend Danny is dead.

"How are you?" I am repeatedly asked by concerned friends.

I don't know. I'm functioning. I think I'm better, but I can't tell for sure. I haven't been to the bathroom in twenty-four hours with any results. What do I say? "I'll let you know when I have a solid bowel movement." Such discourse is not appropriate for a party where food is being served.

Two hours later I have my answer. Hindsight, glorious hindsight, tells me that I shouldn't have gone out for a tuna-salad sandwich after the party.

The tests find nothing, as usual. My doctor tells me that *Giardia* can be missed.

Perhaps it's just a spastic colon.

I have a feeling that I am being shortchanged on my pills. I had a script for two hundred Zovirax and the pharmacy was running low, so it gave me fifty on Friday and I had to pick up the rest on Monday, but on Monday the delivery hadn't come, so the pharmacy gave me another fifty and I picked up one hundred the following day. This didn't involve two extra trips because the first day I was also picking up Mycostatin for my yeast infection, a delicious yogurt-smooth liquid in suspension, which means if I take it to work, chances are it will mess up my backpack. I prefer pills and IV solutions. And on Tuesday I was picking up Flagyl because I still have the runs and I may have *Giardia*. So I went and counted one of the fifty-pill bottles and I only got forty-eight, and I have no idea if this was because I miscounted or because I had already taken a dose of two or if the pharmacist was cheating me. Well, cheating my insurance company, although I do have to pay $7.50 for every prescription, and that means four pills are worth fifteen cents, which might buy a single banana on the street in certain neighborhoods, and of course it means I would have to go to the pharmacy more often, but in fact I'm going so frequently anyway that one more prescription would merely mean I could consolidate my visits.

The pills are a scythe in my belly, a dagger to my heart.

There is a thin metallic taste on everything I ingest.

After a few days of Flagyl, I begin to think I'm losing it. I can no longer shit. Period. Bile is accumulating. It has to have some method of egress. My stomach continues gurgling like a just-opened bottle of Canada Dry ginger ale, my stomach continues roiling like some wide Sargasso Sea. The anal orifice is completely blocked for the time being. Hence, I am left with only one alternative.

To my surprise, suddenly, belief in a higher power returns as I soundlessly retch on hands and knees into the toilet. I realize I am in the bargaining phase of diarrhea. "Please please please let me get better," I plead to some invisible deity or force of logic. "Just let me get better. I promise never to eat anything more complex than bananas or applesauce. Just please let me get better." Rational thought decrees that in order to bargain, a higher power must exist with which to bargain. Perhaps all religions are predicated on bargaining and rational thought. Then I remember: I am an atheist. It is all futile. There is no God. If there was, He died in the first reel, and I have a feeling we're rapidly approaching the Act Two finale.

Could this be the day? I sit on the toilet and imagine myself surrounded by fans, waiting in anticipation. Good or bad? Loose or solid? Aqueous or corklike? Floater or sinker? The buzzer will go off if this specimen fails the rigid criteria and exacting standards of the panel of experts who sit in judgment. I'm a contestant on "Jeopardy!" who has bet everything on that final category, deduced the correct answer, but forgotten to formulate it as a question. I'm approaching an emotional epiphany through the process of elimination.

I flash back to my first bowel movement and potty training.

• • •

"Shall I tell you the consistency of my latest effort?" I ask my friend Wayne, the relentless top and total control freak who giggles incessantly, on the phone.

"I'd be only too delighted to hear it," he replies.

I think of much as I contemplate the tiles on the bathroom floor.

What is the thin line between normal health and HIV? Is this diarrhea that bizarre? Is this something I could have if I were HIV-negative? Am I violently ill, or is it all my imagination, the mental amplification of minor symptoms and ailments to the resonant frequency of insanity? It is getting harder and harder to distinguish between common ailments and pathology.

What separates me from everyone else? Low T-cells? It's just a number. The seventeen thousand and one warts on my hands? I can always wear gloves. An insane fear of death? That's completely normal. The runs? Who doesn't have the runs once in a while? An occasional allergic reaction capable of immobilizing me for a week? I have one friend who gets hives when he eats seafood, and another who has asthma. A ream of prescriptions and monthly doctors' visits? Maybe I'm just a hypochondriac. Fatigue? Is there anyone who lives in New York City who doesn't have at least a mild case of fatigue?

A week later (May 22, 1993) I'm scheduled for one day's worth of community service because I was arrested, along with more than two hundred gay activists, for marching in protest of the Saint Patrick's Day Parade. Peter, Jan, and I have elected against taking the charges to trial because we just don't want to go through the hassle of forty-nine court appearances to have half the charges thrown out as unconstitutional, maybe leaving one charge that sticks, for which we will be required to do three to five days' community service. I have only so much vacation time to take. I keep missing work. One day for the faux flu, another for the turkey trots. I keep taking long lunches for demos. I really didn't plan on getting arrested on Saint Patrick's Day; when I was finally released, I called in to work and said I was "detained."

But I'm worried: How will I last eight hours working in a park without my own personal Portosan? I'm better, but still, I'm not altogether sure. I wake up on Saturday at a quarter to seven so I can meet Jan and Peter for breakfast at seven; we take a cab to the park and get there by eight. Our eight hours of community service shrink to forty-seven minutes of actual work, because the trash compactor broke down after we shoveled some rocks into it. It wasn't *my* idea. The sanitation worker told us to do it.

Now when I am kissed, should I turn my face to the left for a chaste peck on the cheek, like the rest of my terminally ill friends who are afraid of the tiniest bugs? Poor Tim has no short-term memory left at all; Joy had to give him his cha-cha heels seven times last Wednesday in the hospital.

If only I had taken Imodium that first night. If only I had forced myself to vomit immediately and cleared my system of whatever wretched substances it had ingested. If only I called my doctor on the first day. If only I stopped eating freshly grated Romano cheese. If only I took Gas-X on a regular basis. If only I wasn't so high-strung and nervous. If only I knew how to meditate. If only I believed in a higher power. If only.

I like to remember the simple time when life was a series of multiple-choice quizzes, and all I needed for success was a sharpened No. 2 pencil and a uniform standardized-answer sheet. I try to reformulate my new-gained knowledge from this dreadful experience into several basic rules. Hindsight is certainly unfair, but occasionally has some practical value. Through hindsight we are allowed the illusion of correcting the past and preventing calamities in the future.

I am comforted by the fact that I won't have to go through this again, or if I do, at least it will be easier. Yet I know in my heart of hearts that I will—if not this, then some other medical monstrosity. And it will only be worse.

Notes
on
Death

Death means never having to say you're sorry.

Death means never being able to say you're sorry.

Death is not proud.

Death has always relied on the kindness of strangers.

Death wears a herringbone suit, a skinny tie, and a black hat.

Death does not brake for pedestrians.

Death is an equal-opportunity antagonist.

Death does not discriminate.

Death is left-handed.

Death is losing its hair.

Death never needs a face-lift.

Death is frequently played by Max von Sydow on the silver screen.

Death is always in style but never in fashion.

Death wears only black.

Death lives in the East Village.

Death does not have a goatee.

Death can be announced at any location: over meat loaf at a dismal diner; in a hospital waiting room; at an ACT UP political funeral; at the Saint-at-Large New Year's Eve party; at the Trouble party at Zone DK.

Death is the end of all pain.

Death is the end of all pleasure.

Death is the next-best thing to being there.

Death is the final exam, and there are no makeups.

Death can be prematurely embraced as suicide.

Death cannot be cheated.

Death is a way of avoiding responsibilities.

Death masquerades on the subway as a sleeping derelict.

Death does not know the outcome of next year's Academy Awards.

Death is the one thing worse than being stuck on It's a Small, Small World for all eternity.

Death does not take kindly to constructive criticism: Hell hath no greater fury than death scorned.

Death comes in like a lion and goes out like the endless abyss.

You Can't
Wear a Red
Ribbon
If You're
Dead

I'd like to thank the Tony Awards committee and the true husband of my heart—oh, sorry, wrong speech.

I know you're eagerly awaiting those lesbian folk singers from the Soviet Ukraine; please bear with me. The bisexual marching band should be coming in around ten o'clock, and the Gay Caucus for Reasonably Priced Tickets to Bette Midler is auctioning off the only pair of underwear that Sharon Stone has worn in the past three years.

I know I should be talking about the great issues of the day, like whether red ribbons represent a deep-seated commitment to fighting the AIDS epidemic even when they involve color-clashing, or whether they are merely used to express our solidarity with the people who attend the Tony Awards.

I know I should be talking about gays and lesbians in the military. Our grand marshals, Perry Watkins and Miriam Ben-Shalom, are our heroes. And I'm not just saying this because Miriam has me locked in her rifle sights. *Of course* we are opposed

---

Speech delivered at Gay Pride rally, Union Square, New York City, June 26, 1993.

to homophobic discrimination in the military. Everybody here should read Randy Shilts's relentless *Conduct Unbecoming* to find out just how horrifying these witch-hunts have been and continue to be. But we can't afford to lose focus on AIDS. At times the emphasis on the military made the March on Washington feel like the Nuremberg rally to me.

Unfortunately, we have a President who is capable of handling only one lesbian-and-gay-related issue at a time. The military is the sexy issue this year. So it's taken Bill Clinton five fucking months to name an AIDS czar who doesn't report directly to the President or even to the Chief of Staff, but to a domestic-policy adviser. And whatever happened to the Manhattan Project he promised?

I'm halfway down that HIV Highway to Hell. You know the route: Finding out you're positive, telling your friends, your first nucleoside-analogue reverse-transcriptase inhibitor, telling the folks, your second nucleoside-analogue reverse-transcriptase inhibitor, your first bad reaction to a PCP prophylactic, your third nucleoside-analogue reverse-transcriptase inhibitor, telling your prospective tricks, your diagnosis according to the recently changed CDC definition of PWLTC—Person With Lousy T-cells—your fourth nucleoside-analogue reverse-transcriptase inhibitor, telling your current boyfriend, your first infusion, your thirty-ninth arrest with ACT UP, your ninety-third placebo-controlled protocol, your forty-eighth opportunistic infection, and eventually, hopefully after the Oscars, Gay Pride, and Part 2 of *Angels in America,* you achieve the status of metabolically challenged, which is a polite way of saying "dead."

You can't wear a red ribbon if you're dead. You can't march in the Saint Patrick's Day parade if you're dead. You can't register as domestic partners if you're dead. You can't belong to the military if you're dead.

I've been a member of ACT UP since 1987. ACT UP is a diverse, nonpartisan group, united in anger and committed to end-

ing the AIDS crisis. I know, it feels as if the great moment of ACT
UP has passed. Many of our members have burnt out. Many more
have died. After finishing his duties as bus monitor, David Serko
calmly set up his infusion on the bus ride to Kennebunkport
when ACT UP invaded Bush's summer home. David Serko is
dead. Tom Cunningham selflessly managed our work-space for
two years with heart and soul. Tom Cunningham is dead. Katrina
Haslip brought AIDS activism to the New York City prison system. Katrina Haslip is dead. Robert Garcia energized the Latino/
Latina Caucus of ACT UP with his commitment, ideals, and
vitality. Robert Garcia is dead. Last year during the presidential
campaign, Bob Rafsky, our conscience, our reality check, accused
Bill Clinton face to face of dying of ambition while Bob was
dying of AIDS. Bob Rafsky is dead.

It's exhausting fighting this seemingly endless fight. Let's face it:
We're all tired of the AIDS crisis. We're over it. But we're stuck
with it. It's not going away. It might not end in our lifetimes. We
can't just give up. We've got to keep fighting!

If up to half the gay men in New York City are HIV-positive,
can there by any other overriding issue?

Needle-exchange and bleach kits are stopgap measures. Fight
for the Gottfried Bill to decriminalize needles in New York State!
Open the U.S. borders to people who are HIV-positive! We must
never again allow our government to create an HIV concentration
camp, as it did in Guantanamo Bay for Haitian political refugees.
Fight for universal health care and a single-payer system! Managed
care is nothing more than health-care rationing where insurance
companies select your doctors. Teach safer sex and condoms in
schools! The religious Right is literally killing us by ignoring the
realities of teenage sex and preaching only abstinence and blocking education in the public schools. Stop drug companies like
Astra Pharmaceuticals from raping us by charging $30,000 a year
for drugs to fight CMV retinitis! Force drug companies like
Hoffmann–La Roche and Daiichi to stop stonewalling research

on promising drugs for KS and HIV! AIDS is a health crisis, not an opportunity for profit. We need a fully coordinated Manhattan Project to end the AIDS crisis. The Barbara McClintock Project developed by members of ACT UP is one solution. Get President Clinton to fulfill his campaign promises! Fight for the cure! Come to a Monday-night meeting of ACT UP at the Lesbian and Gay Community Services Center.

I'd like to close with a chant.

We will not rest in peace. AIDS CURE NOW!

••

I wrote the first draft of this speech three weeks early and changed it every night, driving Binky crazy. Typically, when I read, it's for a crowd of twenty or thirty. The last time I miscalculated the size of a crowd was that hideous abortion at the New York Public Library where John Weir and I humiliated ourselves in front of four hundred paying guests. We were asked to have a public conversation about using humor in our writing about AIDS. The organizer insisted on a spontaneous exchange. The result was probably no more tedious or embarrassing than the first week of Chevy Chase's canceled talk show.

"They're not going to release the refugees from Guantanamo before Saturday?" I asked my friend Jan.

"Of course not." They did.

"Wayne, Clinton has spent the last six months not naming an AIDS czar. He's not about to name one before Saturday, is he?" I asked on Wednesday.

"It's pretty doubtful."

I gave my friend Terry Callaghan a copy of the speech because he had to work on Saturday. "Oh, Clinton named an AIDS czar today; you'll have to change it."

I was still madly editing the day of the speech. Wayne and Jan had brunch with me so I wouldn't have to be nervous alone. Binky was home making strawberry monstrosities. "He made me clean the tiles on the bathroom floor," I pouted. "Doesn't he understand? Not today." Binky had invited twenty people over after the rally for a strawberry feast.

I was scheduled to speak at 2:15. When I arrived at ten minutes to 2, I was informed that I had been bumped to 5:20. Three more hours to get nervous. I spent maybe fifteen minutes backstage before I spoke. I hurriedly crossed out the references to the hours of guilt-tripping that awaited the attendees. Perry Watkins and Miriam Ben-Shalom sat on lawn furniture and chatted with friends, eating sandwiches. I hoped they would disappear by the time I spoke.

Thanks to my friend Alessandro, "You Can't Wear a Red Ribbon If You're Dead" became a sound bite. All summer long, ACT UP recruitment posters were wheat-pasted throughout the Village and Chelsea. I felt like Tama Janowitz for a brief, fleeting moment. Everywhere I went, I saw my words.

Death
before
Forty

AZT is over in a big way. Put your Burroughs Wellcome blue-caps next to your Nehru jacket and last year's bleeding-heart tattoo. The big fashion statement of 1993, the latest in antiretroviral nucleoside analogues, is d4T. d4T comes in tiny, tastefully subdued industrial-gray logo-less capsules. Echoing the theme of uncertainty in this chaotic world, d4T is available through expanded access only in the Mystery Dose. For that personal touch, d4T is packaged in plain white-plastic bottles, hand-labeled with a unique identifier, label code, patient number, and lot number. I am patient D03952. At the top of the label I am admonished in reversed script to "Return this package and any unused medicine." Two cylindrical silica-gel moisture-absorbent caps marked "Do not eat" are buried in the sea of gray.

After failing AZT (dropping T cells), ddI (neuropathy), and ddC (neuropathy again), my doctor has enrolled me in an expanded-access trial of d4T. It's a good thing the pills are tiny, because I am instructed to take four pills twice a day. There are two doses in this doubly blind protocol. I imagine my blindfolded doctor receiving one month's supply of pharmaceuticals from a blindfolded woman bearing scales who looks suspiciously like the image of Justice in a back alley behind the smoking chimney stacks of a multinational drug company somewhere in South Jersey. d4T is the fourth Drug for Testing in the nucleoside-analogue sequence. Subconsciously, it echoes the antithesis of one of my increasingly unrealistic goals: Death by Forty. When I attend those discouraging presentations on what we learned from the Berlin AIDS Conference, I find myself dispirited to hear my recent T-cell counts (in the neighborhood of 100) referred to as late-stage disease and severely immunocompromised. Chris DeBlasio, a friend I had met in Ty's four or five years ago when we were both trying to pick up the same Floridian blond who worked at AT&T, was a personal point of inspiration and confidence to me as someone who had been in the 100 T-cell range for years with few or no ill effects. Alas. This last year was brutal to Chris, and he died two weeks ago. And now I find myself inching toward my goal of lasting until forty with somewhat less confidence. Would it be more prudent to plan a ridiculously retro fortieth birthday party complete with ABBA covers on the stereo, a bartender in a leather vest, and pink streamers, or should I spend my time planning my own memorial service?

d4T has the usual side effects: pancreatitis, liver dysfunction, and reversible neuropathy. "It's not always reversible," warns my friend Clay from San Francisco, a divine nephrologist who examined Ferdinand Marcos's kidneys weeks before he died. A shirtless photo of Clay leaning from a branch of a tree advertised some sex service every week in the pages of the *Bay Area Reporter*. After "a tiny bout" of PCP last year, Clay's gym days are over. Pulitzer Prize—winning Paul takes five pills in the morning and three at night, because he finds that d4T keeps him up at night. I have no worries about disturbing my sleep patterns. They've been shot to hell for years.

Sure enough, after one month of d4T, my T-cells are up.

My father referred to the danger signals on a car's dashboard as "idiot lights": By the time they turned on, any damage to the car was irreversible. I found this out in high school when I took Laura E. Grossman to Saratoga Springs and I filled the carburetor with water because the engine was running hot.

The idiot lights in my metabolism have been burning bright for years.

Unfortunately, I run out of pills at the end of the month, and have to wait four days for the next supply. d4T isn't available at your friendly pharmacist's counter. The local buyers' club doesn't stock it. You can't buy it on the street at black-market rates.

A month later, in a move calculated only to irritate me, my doctor's receptionist calls me at home on Friday while I'm at work, to announce that my shipment of d4T has arrived. This is similar to getting a yellow slip at 1:05 on Saturday afternoon that they have a package for me at the local post office, which closed at 1:00 P.M., and Monday is a federal holiday; consequently, I have to wait until Tuesday to pick up that special item from International Male that doesn't fit anyway.

The first Friday in July, having returned from Tim Bailey's aborted political funeral in D.C., I have another message on my machine concerning d4T. I assume that my new supply is at the office. I have enough for the weekend, so I don't bother calling back. On Monday I'm too busy playing catch-up at work to call; on Tuesday I find out that my liver enzymes have gone through the roof, from 20 to 200. I must stop d4T immediately. Last Thursday by the earliest. I'm tempted to celebrate. My doctor warned me against any alcohol. Which is why you'll find me at the Break that night at midnight, sitting in front of six empty glasses that formerly contained Shirley Temples.

At the GMHC/TAG/CRIA forum on the Berlin AIDS Conference, I hear good news and bad news. The bad news is that nucleoside analogues aren't that good; the good news is that now doctors are telling their asymptomatic patients that they will support whatever treatment decisions the patient makes, including no treatment. Nucleoside analogues like AZT seem to be of limited effectiveness for a small window of opportunity; as for me, I've already jumped years ago. The good news is these relatively ineffective pills aren't as toxic as previously feared.

Two weeks later I give my doctor another fifteen pints of blood. While I'm there, he checks my lungs, my feet, and gives me a B shot. The following day he tells me my counts are back to normal, and I should restart the d4T, this time taking two pills twice a day. I should see him in another two weeks for another blood test.

My feet start tingling in two days. This worrisome symptom comes and goes; it's worst when I wake up. I'm not really sure, but I think it's neuropathy. I decide to stop the d4T.

In the past three weeks, Jon Greenberg, David Kirschenbaum, and Chris DeBlasio have died.

I feel guilty. Neuropathy is so sketchy. How do I tell my doctor? I feel I haven't done my best for science. I would gladly donate a few lymph nodes and withstand several months of minor pain, maybe even a nice scar, in the cause of scientific progress. Yesterday's *Times* had a human-interest story about a subject on the three-pronged antiretroviral protocol. Last February a group of researchers announced that they had found "what may be the Achilles' heel" of the virus in laboratory tests. It turns out the researchers were the heels. Yet this subject wasn't dropping out of the protocol because the theoretical underpinnings of the trial had been blown to pieces. He had a severely damaged immune system, according to the article, and his T-cells were 552, up from 414. I would kill to be at that level. At that moment I wanted to destroy every laboratory test that I've taken in the past six years.

I remember a time in the early sixties when the future was bright, science was a virtue, and progress was another step toward utopia. The space program had already brought us Tang, the instant powdered citrus beverage, and Space Food sticks in aluminum wrappers. Products gleamed with brightly colored contrasting patches of "NEW!" "IMPROVED!" "PROTEIN-FORTIFIED!" What would we do without chemicals? Anything was possible if you just added water.

The more technical the name of the scientific compound, the more promising it appeared to be to me. Burroughs Wellcome's 566C80 not only kept PCP at bay, it actually killed the organism, at least in the test tube. Now that it has been approved with the boring name Mepron, it isn't half as effective as I had hoped it would be.

Understand that I'm biting my tongue as I say the following: **AZT is shit. ddC is shit. ddI is shit. d4T is shit.**

Honey, I'm over these nucleoside analogues. Can we try something else now, please?

Keep the date November 25, 1996, open. I am still planning on having that fortieth-birthday party, come hell or high water. At this point, I fully expect it to be a huge bonfire on the lawn of the White House. I'll be there. Let's all join hands and form a circle around my funeral pyre for progress.

The
Gastronomic
Me

It is six in the morning on a school day in June 1993 and I'm lying on the bathroom floor, curled up in the fetal position, clutching the throw-carpet to my breast, and wondering whether I have a ruptured spleen, appendicitis, or an ulcer. Is it a peptic ulcer? Is it a duodenal ulcer? Or is it merely gastric acid from hell? I anxiously thumb through my mass-market paperback edition of *Man's Body: An Owner's Manual* for hints and suggestions. If I am going to spend the rest of my life in the bathroom, I should probably unearth that spare phone from the storage cabinet and plug it into the jack next to the toilet for the ultimate in meaningless glamour. Binky plods in (pat, pat, pat) and asks, concerned, "Are you okay?"

I croak, "Not really," and he returns to bed (pat, pat, pat) as I lie collapsed in a heap on the bathroom floor, wondering when it will end.

This is my fifth attack. Each usually lasts one hour and then after I've lost all hope it gradually dissipates (thanks, perhaps, to the tablet of Pepto-Bismol I've taken, or the Maalox mint). It starts with a sharp pain in my stomach. My entire torso is racked with discomfort, as if I've pulled every single muscle from an overly optimistic workout. The pressure is such that I cannot think, I cannot rest. Once I tried a bath: If I immersed myself in water, perhaps I would feel weightless. It worked for exactly five minutes. I try to remember the last thing I ingested. A glass of orange juice. Too bitter? Too sour? What exactly is the cause of these attacks? Is it anxiety? If so, why wasn't I born with this? Could it have anything to do with the minor domestic squabbles I have with my boyfriend an average of four times a day?

I find myself becoming a parody of everything I've read or seen. I am Portnoy's father, sitting on the toilet for an hour every night, reading the obituaries. I am the Mormon in *Angels in America* who takes a Pepto-Bismol chaser after a slug of Coke. But, worse, I am my own father, who died at the age of fifty-two, sitting up in bed and clutching his chest at five in the morning, thinking it was heartburn when it was actually a heart attack.

Damn. I already wrote my fucking speech for Gay Pride, three weeks in advance, so instead of procrastinating and agonizing about it every night in the abstract and having nightmares about standing in front of ten thousand people naked without a speech, I could constantly revise it and agonize about it every night in the concrete and have nightmares about sitting in the emergency room as they announce me at the rally. My doctor is off in Vienna or Amsterdam or Berlin, at another international AIDS conference. Why bother doing *anything* in advance? What's the point of standing in line for half an hour to get tickets to Bette Midler's concert in September and then finding out they take only cash and then going to the cash machine and then going to another outlet that is closed for lunch and then returning to Tower Records and finally getting tickets, when I may not even make it and I might have to give them away, or, worse yet, waste them?

Today was the day I was finally going to finish Randy Shilts's epic saga of betrayal, *Conduct Unbecoming,* and maybe start something easier like *War and Peace.* Today was the day I was going to do twenty-four minutes on the Stair Master at the highest setting.

Today was the day I was going to finish my play, work on the novel that has been on hold since a year ago November, and sketch out a few more essays. But it looks as if I'll spend most of the day on the bathroom floor.

There is no blood in my stool. There is no stool. I want to vomit but I can't. The best I can manage is to cough. I go to the living room to lie on the couch, and my boyfriend plods into the bathroom (pat, pat, pat), uses the toilet (flush!), and goes back to bed (pat, pat, pat). The cause of his concern reveals itself to me. I can't lie on the couch. I go to bed and try to lie down. I can't. I get up and walk around. And gradually it goes away.

I go back to bed and caress Binky's back. He groans in his sleep and greets my touch with affection and rolls over and begins snoring. Perhaps the most successful moments of our relationship occur when one or both of us is unconscious. I decide to set my alarm for later to make up for the missing hour of sleep.

"You would know if you had appendicitis," says my friend Tom later that day. "Your appendix is on the right, halfway between your dick and your belly button." But I'm left-handed. Maybe it's transposed.

After my last attack, I was convinced I had developed a highly specific allergy to freshly grated Pecorino Romano cheese. I had had two attacks after eating pasta. It could have been the sauce; it could have been the pasta. But I had ceremoniously thrown out the sauce. It lay in the trash, next to the mocha-fudge cake that rose only two centimeters because as usual I got some yolk in the egg white and didn't whisk it for twenty-four hours so it would be hard and fluffy and my boyfriend found the frosting too sweet and it ended up in the trash in a minor hissy fit after I guess we had another minor domestic squabble when he came home to find me watching the Tony Awards and clutching a friend, but not the friend he expected.

• • •

A week later I have another attack just as I am about to leave for work. I call in semi-sick; I figure I'll be in later. I figure maybe my stomach is empty, a vat of boiling acid, screaming, "Feed me! Feed me!" I eat a piece of bread and swallow a cup of milk. I throw it up in the toilet. I rest. I wait. Sure enough, an hour later, maybe a little queasy, maybe a little weak, I'm ready to roll to work. Cautiously I order a mocha-almond muffin at Michael's Muffins. Five minutes in the door at work and I'm back in the bathroom, throwing up mocha. I clutch my legs at the ankles. All color leaches from my face. I limp back to my office and shut the door. I take several deep breaths. I send Terry C. out on a mission of mercy: Mylanta. I reschedule my Tuesday appointment for 2:30 P.M. I wait.

It's not an ulcer. It's not colitis. It's not kidney stones. It's not appendicitis.

It's gas. Gas in my colon.

My doctor recommends Mylanta Gas or Gas-X, three or four times a day. "Relieves gas pain, pressure, and bloating," according to the package insert. Plain Mylanta might cause diarrhea.

Once again I feel like a capital I Idiot.

Gas. That's it?

He tells me to avoid carbonated beverages. I practically live on Canada Dry seltzer. My options are already grossly limited when it comes to barroom fare. Beer is already off the list. A single beer will give me indigestion for the night. You might as well forget hard liquor completely. I used to think it was ludicrous to order seltzer at a bar. At least beer has some substance. Seltzer is free from the spritzer. I know, I was brought up cheap. Now scratch the simple carbonated beverages, including soda water. Now I can't even order Shirley Temples. I guess I'm stuck with cranberry-juice cocktails and other assorted citrus juices.

He also says avoid yeasty foods. Watch out for beer, onions, and beans. Eat yogurt. He won't prescribe cramp medicine, because by the time it takes effect, my attack is over anyway.

What am I left with? Is cheese good or bad? Should I avoid citrus and tomato products? Will my stomach ever regain its flatness? My choices are limited. I feel like a cow, producing enough methane from my four stomachs to raise the temperature of the planet five degrees. How do you remove gas from gastronomy?

Three weeks later, when my liver enzymes go through the roof as a possible side effect of d4T, my doctor casually suggests that this may have played a role in my gastric discomfort of the past.

Six weeks later the city declares a water emergency in my neighborhood. Don't drink from the tap! By the time I make it over to the local D'Agostino, there's nothing left but a couple of six packs of 11.2-ounce bottles of Evian at $4.49. I buy two.

I decide I'm over tap water, carbonated beverages, and nucleoside analogues. I have had some rather unpleasant nights due to eating fried food after eleven, but cross my fingers, no stomach-clutching attacks since then.

Perhaps I spoke too soon. For most of August, I've awakened every night at approximately 3:15 A.M. for an urgent bathroom visit, which, more likely than not, will consist purely of air. After, I lie down. A rock is anchored at the base of my stomach. I turn to my side. I lie on my stomach. I mimic an advanced position from Twister, arms splayed and legs crossed, in an attempt to find a comfortable position. My center of gravity is out of kilter. The rock weighs me down. I feel dizzy and mildly nauseated.

Some nights I try another Mylanta Gas, or a few swigs of Mylanta. Some nights I take an Ativan. Some nights I twist and moan until dawn, without ever losing consciousness.

My doctor offered the new! improved! take-home stool test. I produce samples at 1:15 A.M. and 2:30 A.M., which I store on the condiment shelf of the refrigerator. I take a cab to the lab the next morning. I discover I need to produce one more sample. I find the greasiest spoon in ten blocks and order the special. Twenty minutes later, I am back at the lab.

A week later I find out that I am parasite-free. My doctor gives me a daily ulcer pill, which doesn't seem to work. "Are there any foods that seem to irritate you particularly?"

"Everything," I reply.

"Maybe it's your gallbladder. Try a low-fat diet."

There is something suspiciously random about this. I imagine my doctor pulling down an anatomical flip-chart hinged on springs, then tossing a dart at it at random, only to find it land on the gallbladder.

I have always produced phenomenal amounts of gas, but only recently has my alimentary canal developed a few new cul-de-sacs, and there is no easy method of egress anymore. Perhaps a simple chiropractic session would straighten me out? Perhaps a plumber's helper?

I easily spend entire nonproductive afternoons at my office hunched over my desk, half-asleep from the previous night, attempting casually to reshuffle the paperwork should someone enter the door with more mail. It's only a matter of time before I get caught.

Ethical
Suicide Alternatives

Or, How to Get Someone Else to
Do the Job for You

The implements of violent death must be in plain view and easily accessible even to the most obtuse and physically unfit. A loaded gun is best. It is helpful to have handy a pair of gloves of appropriate size, along with a lint-free cloth to wipe off fingerprints. A plastic bag from the cleaner's should be accompanied by a length of rope or wire, a telephone cord, or a heavy-duty rubber band. Butcher's knives are generally too messy, and require an unnecessary amount of personal involvement.

It is best not to wait until you are hospitalized. Some of the following plans require considerable time and preparation. They may be impossible to implement from a hospital bed. Furthermore, members of the medical profession who have taken the Hippocratic oath have a tendency to attempt to revive you.

Keep in mind that the best plan is the simplest. Complicated long-range plans may not succeed. You may not have the luxury of time. On the other hand, simply letting nature take its course is ultimately the most effective, albeit frustrating, method.

1. Invite all of his exes to a cocktail party and surprise him.
2. Certain albums, such as Bob Dylan's *Self-Portrait,* the

251

252 •••••••• LIFE IN HELL

soundtrack to *The Coneheads*, or anything by Andrew Lloyd Webber, can do the trick. Personal taste here counts mightily; some people, although invulnerable to show tunes, will find operatic arias intolerable. It helps if the doors are locked and there is no easy method of egress.

3. Casually mention to him that you've tricked with his ostensibly monogamous lover of seventeen years. You may find it necessary to add that you think the condom may have broken. As a coup de grace, try: "That's funny, I got hepatitis, too, around the time Ernie got it last summer." Then blush profusely and attempt lamely to change the subject.

4. Ply her with high-caloric junk food, such as Hostess Twinkies.

5. Have an ill-advised affair with him. Break it off abruptly. Call up his machine nightly and play Whitney Houston's rendition of "I Will Always Love You" in its entirety.

6. Timing can be everything. Pay particular attention to high-stress periods in his or her life: career pressure points, mid-life crises, and sudden dietary changes. Be sure to chart his or her biorhythms, astrological sign, and menstrual cycle.

7. Give him an unrecoverably bad haircut under sedation before a public testimonial dinner involving his parents, his high-school drama teacher, and his boss.

8. Tickle him until he loses control of his bladder on his brand-new Persian rug that cost more than four months' salary.

9. Put arsenic in his fish tank. Shoot up his cat with heroin. Feed cocaine to his parakeet. Put his poodle in the microwave. Marinate his pet iguana overnight in a basil-and-salsa sauce and feed it to him as a cocktail appetizer. Kill his dog. Feed his parrot to his cat. Sexually abuse his gerbils. Leave a discreet note of apology on the bureau.

10. Masturbate on the white-linen Armani suit he recently scored from Barneys' Labor Day sale.

11. Discuss certain of his more arcane sexual practices with his mother.

12. Invite him over for Sunday brunch. Feed him a delicious spinach-and-bacon salad with clams *oreganata*. Slip a few laxatives into the brownies. Call to tell him about your amoebas the following Tuesday.

13. Borrow his videocassette of the Tonys and tape "Married with Children" over it.

14. Order any twelve items from the latest Undergear catalog to be sent to his address under his name. A discreet inquiry a few months later will confirm that it was you.

15. Get involved in a summer share with him on Fire Island and be yourself. This is the slowest, but surest, solution. I guarantee he will kill you, if you haven't killed him first.

Political
Funerals

I imagine what it would be like if friends had a demonstration each time a lover or a friend or a stranger died of
AIDS. I imagine what it would be like if, each time a lover,
friend or stranger died of this disease, their friends, lovers or
neighbors would take the dead body and drive with it in a
car a hundred miles an hour to washington d.c. and blast
through the gates of the white house and come to a screeching halt before the entrance and dump their lifeless form on
the front steps.

—David Wojnarowicz,
Close to the Knives

This past year, it seems that ACT UP is coming to terms with death.

David Robinson initiated the Ashes Action from San Francisco.
His lover, Warren, had died that past spring. At first David was
thinking of mailing Warren's ashes to the White House as a private
gesture of anger, grief, and protest. Upon reflection, he decided a
public forum would be more appropriate. There was strong sup-

port for the concept of an ashes action on the floor of ACT UP/N.Y. The Names Quilt was going to be displayed for the last time in its entirety in Washington, D.C., during Columbus Day weekend in October 1992. We decided to have the demonstration on Sunday of that weekend. We were going to shower the White House lawn with the ashes of our loved ones.

I remember seeing Warren and David dance together in a bar in Atlanta, when ACT UP/N.Y. flew down for a series of demonstrations against the CDC and the sodomy laws. Warren was gorgeous. He wore a white tank top. David Robinson had been a facilitator for the Monday-night ACT UP meetings for several years. He frequently came to meetings in postmodern drag: a skirt and a beard. David was a trained dancer. He was strong and passionate.

Warren was from the South. David and Warren moved together to San Francisco, shortly after David, as one of the "Three Anonymous Queers," penned the broadside "I Hate Straights." Warren and David were a discordant couple: Warren was positive and David was negative. After they moved to San Francisco, I heard only infrequent reports through thirdhand sources about them. Someone told me that Warren had flown to Switzerland for Dr. Roka's herb-enema treatment. My friend Sarah told me it did wonders for her friend Bo. Bo died this spring.

As time passed, more people joined the Ashes Action. They, too, were committed to bringing the ashes of their loved ones to the White House. Shane Butler coordinated the action from New York. We had a series of pre-action meetings. We formed affinity groups to march in rows at the action. Our basic objective was to protect those carrying ashes from the police until they reached the White House. My affinity group was willing to risk arrest.

We felt it wasn't our action, it was David's action, and the action of those carrying ashes of friends and companions. We were merely functioning as support. We decided to have a large, silent, dignified procession to the White House.

That Sunday, we meet at the Capitol side of the Mall. We march down the Mall to the accompaniment of the saddest drums. At first it is just the few busloads of activists from New York and the small group of maybe ten people carrying ashes. As we march silently, people join in from the sidelines. The procession grows. We are silent, for once. SILENCE = DEATH is a metaphor, after all. This is no metaphor: We carry death itself.

Frank, an activist now living in the Midwest, had smeared his face with fake blood and was chanting loudly. "It's not just their demo, it's all of us," he says when reprimanded to be quiet. David wails. Suddenly those carrying the ashes begin to chant. We all chant to the beat of the drums.

As the procession veers north from the Mall to the street, my affinity group functions as the front guard, risking arrest. We pass the pressure point unscathed.

It is impossible for me to assimilate this as it is happening. It is too immense. Our grief is literal. Does a man cease to become more than a symbol after he is dead? Yet somehow this is more than the usual "cheap theatrics," more than our street theater with strong graphics and media savvy.

A woman hands a bag of ashes, her son's, to someone as we march by. She wanted someone to use it. The crowd continues to grow, until we are almost four hundred.

We march in strength and solidarity.

We march in anger and in grief.

We march against the murderous neglect of two presidential administrations.

We march in dignity and pride.

When there is no possibility of getting to the front of the White House, we march to the backyard. The police cluster around on horses. They are planning on stopping us at the end of the driveway, before the fence.

Every action has one mad moment of uncertainty, one delirious moment of fear. We break ranks and make a mad rush, surrounding those carrying the ashes. Mounted policemen move in, forming a wedge between the group at the fence and the group on the other side of the macadam. We sit down to hold our ground. I look down and see a puddle of blood. For a moment I am hysterical. Then I realize it is more of Frank's fake blood.

Some scale the fences and start dumping their containers of ashes, to cheers. And then it is all over.

The police threaten to arrest all those on the fence side of their line. Another gauntlet is thrown. We confer and decide that we've accomplished what we came for and there is no sense in getting arrested after achieving our goal. We will disperse in groups.

We gather in the park behind the White House for a public speak-out. People tell what had happened. I learn of Alexis's grief: She had carried her father's ashes, her father who had died several years ago, and now she is finally experiencing a sense of closure. Eric Sawyer has Larry Kert's celebrity ashes. Larry was disinvited from the White House after he came down with AIDS. Well, now he's coming, invitation or not. David talks about Warren. He cries. And suddenly it rains in torrents, an intense downpour of grief. We rush to a covered grandstand at the side of the park, soaked. The ashes mix with the soil. Ten minutes earlier the Parks Service could have cleaned up our burnt offerings with ease. Now they are impossible to eradicate.

The last time I saw Mark Fisher alive was at Tim Powers's memorial. He was much thinner than I remembered. Mark was an architect from Iowa and a member of The Marys affinity group. He silk-screened T-shirts for The Marys that said "ALL PEOPLE WITH AIDS ARE INNOCENT." Mark was tall and lanky. If Eddie Haskell were gay, he would have grown up to be Mark Fisher.

For three years I sat next to Mark Bronnenberg at ACT UP meetings. He was the other Mark from Iowa. He moved to San Francisco a few years ago, as did Pam and Russell. Pam and Russell were Mark Fisher's best friends. Pam's brother died of

AIDS. Pam was very hurt when the "I Hate Straights" broadsheet came out.

Mark Fisher wrote an anonymous piece published by *QW* a few weeks before his death titled "Bury Me Furiously." I'll quote the last section here:

> I suspect—I know—my funeral will shock people when it happens. We Americans are terrified of death. Death takes place behind closed doors and is removed from reality, from the living. I want to show the reality of my death, to display my body in public; I want the public to bear witness. We are not just spiraling statistics; we are people who have lives, who have purpose, who have lovers, friends, and families. And we are dying of a disease maintained by a degree of criminal neglect so enormous that it amounts to genocide.
>
> I want my death to be as strong a statement as my life continues to be.
>
> I want my own funeral to be fierce and defiant, to make the public statement that my death from AIDS is a form of political assassination.
>
> We are taking this action out of love and rage.

It is all so very terrible. Mark died of sepsis, caused by a catheter infection, on the plane coming back from Italy, less than a month after the Ashes Action. He went to Italy with Russell. During the last few days of their vacation, they were looking at hospitals. Mark was going crazy. He kept a diary. The last entry, on the morning of his death, in tiny, tiny writing, was: "Mind is clear. Feel like a complete whole." The last thing he said to Russell was "Hello." Why does dying on a plane freak me out so much?

Mark Fisher was so sweet. I tried calling Mark Bronnenberg in San Francisco three times to let him know. I found out he had died on Thursday, the day after Paul's memorial, the afternoon I found out that Richard was dead.

On Friday there is a Take Back the Night march through the East Village, sponsored by Outwatch and the Anti-Violence Project. It starts at Cooper Union. The mood is grim: Everyone is finding out that Mark Fisher had died. The Marys pass out flyers with Mark's picture on the front, and "Bury Me Furiously" on the back. There will be a political funeral next Monday, the day before the presidential election. Tom came to the demo late. He had to see Luis, who is dying of leukemia, and then his friend Chris had a hissy fit because Tom was a half hour late and Barry blurted out to Tom, "Did you hear that Mark died?" There are times when I cannot comprehend what is going on. There is too much sadness in the world. I suppose Pam knew. Russell must have told her.

I am living under a heavy sheet of sadness.

On Monday there is a ceremony at Judson Memorial Church at Washington Square. Pam has flown in from San Francisco. Russell is there in the front row, with Pam. Afterward, six people carry Mark's open casket up Sixth Avenue to Republican National Headquarters in midtown. His pale and emaciated corpse is clearly visible in the plain-pine coffin. It is raining steadily. The street is a sea of black umbrellas. A car follows the procession. James, on crutches, rides in the car for several blocks. Four people carry burning torches. I am a marshal assigned to the back of the march. I have to make sure that nobody lags behind and is picked off by police.

How many more have to die?

There is some heckling from the sidelines. Police block traffic for us. Sixth Avenue becomes a huge traffic jam. To the passengers in the cars, the drivers, the people walking home in the rain, this is a minor annoyance, just one more aggravation for living in New York. To us, a life, a death. A man on the north side of Washington Square Park yells at us, thinking it is just another pro-Clinton demonstration. It doesn't sink in. I am furious, screaming at passersby, "This is a fucking funeral, don't you get it?"

We reach our destination and have a brief ceremony. The door to the building is double-locked. People are hiding from us. Michael Cunningham speaks eloquently and angrily at the end of the procession. The casket is loaded into the car. We leave our list of demands at Republican headquarters, the same list of demands we left at Kennebunkport a year ago. These are the same demands we keep on pressing: Open the borders to HIV-positives. Distribute condoms in the schools. Fund needle-exchange programs throughout the country. Have a massive research project to find a cure for AIDS. Double the NIH budget. Put someone in charge of the crisis.

We go home. What have we accomplished? Are we any closer to ending this crisis?

Tim Bailey wanted us to throw his body over the White House fence, but we couldn't do that—"not because we didn't share his fury but because we loved him too much to treat his mortal remains that way," as Michael Cunningham said at his memorial. Instead, we chartered two buses and drove to D.C. at seven-thirty in the morning. Without a second thought, one hundred activists take off work Thursday to go to a political funeral to honor Tim Bailey. I can't sleep the night before. I am up at six. On the way down to Washington, a video on AIDS activism plays on the monitor. I huddle next to my friend Brian and try to get some sleep.

Tim was a fashion designer for the house of Patricia Field. James Baggett and Joy were his best friends. Tim was a frail bleach-blond. He had been ill for more than a year. Last summer I saw him on Fire Island. He was there for a weekend with Joy and her girlfriend. He confessed to Michael Cunningham that Fire Island was the only place on earth he truly felt safe. He had grown up to the taunt "faggot." Even in New York City, it was difficult to escape the homophobia of this culture.

We arrive in D.C. at noon. We mill around for an hour, trying not to look too conspicuous. We fail. One hundred activists with ACT UP T-shirts, stickers, and posters can't exactly fade into the reflecting pool by the Capitol. Some of us have pinned Tim Bailey's photo to our chests. Some have drums.

An hour later the van arrives with Tim's body. Several police cars have appeared in the interim. We are told to gather away from the van to form the procession. A few minutes later we hear there is trouble.

The police won't let us remove the casket from the van.

The police tell us to move away from the back of the van. We surge there and recapture our ground. Two lone police officers from the back of the van, feeling the crush of fifty activists, excuse themselves and make their exits.

This begins a three-hour standoff.

There are D.C. police, county police, federal police, and police from the Parks Service. We are simultaneously in several jurisdictions and no one is in charge. No officer is able to explain why we are being forbidden to remove the casket. A policeman has the keys to the van. He had wrestled them away from Joy during the initial confrontation. A car is parked in front of the van, blocking it.

Then we are told we need a death certificate, and the body must be examined by a coroner, in order to have a procession. The police have to make sure that Tim's death was not a homicide. Even then the police may not allow a procession. There is an arcane regulation that forbids unseemly displays.

Feeling we have made all the proper preparations, feeling we are on the right side of the law, feeling there is some respect for the sanctity of human life, we allow the police to perpetrate this humiliating charade of justice and procedure.

Joy makes the officer come to the coffin. She refuses to let the death certificate out of her hands. She demands and receives back the van keys.

The medical examiner from the coroner's office, wearing rubber gloves, examines the body. Joy and others taunt him as he performs his task. He is close to tears by the time he leaves. "Are you satisfied? Is he dead enough? This is what AIDS looks like. Are you proud of yourself?"

After the police examine the death certificate and the body has been examined, they confer and decide they still will not allow the procession to take place, on the grounds that it is an unseemly and obscene display.

In a way, the police are right.

Death is unseemly.

Death is obscene.

Death is ugly.

A light rain is falling. We haven't eaten since seven o'clock in the morning.

For close to three hours we have stood, we have sat, we have guarded the van holding the body of our friend Tim Bailey as a solid wall of police lines the perimeter of our group. We are in a parking lot. A car blocks us at the front. The cops want us to leave, but there is no possible method of egress available, even if we wanted to go.

There are ongoing negotiations. Eric Sawyer calls Bob Hattoy in the White House on his cellular phone. Someone else calls an official in the Department of Health and Human Services. Permits are waived. We are eventually offered a compromise march. We can follow the vehicle as long as we keep the casket in the van. We will be able to march with the casket for a block, two blocks away from the White House. Then we must return.

We had planned on having a ceremony at the front of the White House and leaving. We would have been long gone if the police had allowed us to proceed when we arrived. Tim's brother, Randy, is consulted. He is appalled. Eventually we accept the compromise. Perhaps we will continue with the procession after the block. Perhaps we won't. We decide that this will be the best way to proceed. We are tired and angry and hurt.

Then, as we are about to start, at three-thirty, after two and a half hours of unpleasantness and ugliness, the police change their mind. We can proceed if we wait until six-thirty, after rush hour.

The police have not acted in an honorable fashion.

The police have just been stalling us for the past three hours.

We decide to take the coffin out of the van and start our procession.

We are operating on the basic assumption that the police will respect the sanctity of death.

We are wrong.

I move with several people on the left side of the van, to give enough room to open the back door of the van. I am face to face with the cops. We open the door and several people start to take out the coffin.

"Put it back in!" scream the police. "Put it back in!"

It seems that they are afraid of death; they are that afraid of the physical evidence of the notorious neglect of this administration and the previous two presidential administrations. Tim Bailey's body is the smoking gun of the epidemic. Tim Bailey's body accuses them of murder with quiet fury.

What follows is one of the most horrible moments of my life. In a fracas that reminds me of *Day of the Locust,* police and pallbearers struggle with the coffin. I can't tell whether the police are trying to shove the coffin back into the van or steal it as evidence of our transgression. This moment of madness is captured on CNN. I can see the coffin banged on the edges. In the extreme violence of the scene, I have the impression that the wood is chipping, splintering, cracking, and breaking. To protect the body, the pallbearers return the coffin to the van. When it is over, the police have arrested Randy Bailey, brother of the deceased, for assaulting a police officer.

Randy Bailey isn't an activist. He isn't a member of ACT UP. He's had no experience with AIDS activism. He's never been arrested for a political protest. Randy Bailey is a straight man from Ohio whose brother died of AIDS.

Someone yells, "Someone volunteer to get arrested with him so he won't be alone!"

I look around. I am tired. Jim Aquino pauses, then marches

straight into the police, and they immediately arrest him. He is as innocent as a lamb led to the slaughter. Two others attempt to get arrested. James Learned tries to break through a solid line of police with the fury of a caged bull, but they won't let him through. He is furious.

This is not a game. This is life and death. This is murder. This is the physical evidence. This is AIDS. This is the remains of Timothy Bailey, dead of AIDS at thirty-five.

We begin our ceremony, on top of the van. Someone sets up the sound system. Several people speak eloquently. Joy is fire and anger.

I cannot speak.

The body is to be returned to the funeral home in New Jersey. Barbara starts the van. The police allow us to have a brief procession out of the parking lot. We march and chant behind the coffin. I stand right behind the van. I do not want the police any closer; I do not want them to have any contact with the van. They desecrate everything they touch. The coffin is surrounded by bouquets of flowers from the funeral home. Jim Baggett starts passing back flowers from the van. Tim used to fill his backpack with flowers on Gay Pride Day and pass out flowers to everyone he saw. In his honor, we pass flowers back until each of us has a flower. At the end of the driveway, the cops push us all aside and form a line between us and the van. Vincent was going to be dropped off at a D.C. hotel with the sound equipment. The police tell them to dump Vincent and the sound equipment on the street. The police give the van an escort all the way to Baltimore, Maryland.

Throughout the entire standoff, an officer stands to the side with a shit-eating grin on his face. "Don't you understand, this is a funeral? Wouldn't you give this much respect to any warrior who died fighting bravely? He's dead! Show some respect!" I am close to hysterical. Barry is infuriated. He wants to go to D.C. the next time a policeman dies in the line of duty to laugh at the funeral service.

• • •

What do you plan on doing with your body after your death? Do you want your body burned in effigy at the offices of the Pharmaceutical Manufacturers Association? Do you want it impaled on the White House fence as an indictment of the current administration? Do you want to donate your HIV-infected organs to the Archdiocese of New York, members of the religious Right, militant antiabortionists, members of the National Rifle Association, feminists against pornography, and right-wing Republicans?

I stand in awe of those like Mark Lowe Fisher and Tim Bailey who are able to commit their bodies for political funerals.

The concept is unfathomable, incomprehensible, as difficult to grasp as death.

Death
Be Not
Proud

It's your best friend Howard's thirty-third birthday, and judging from his recent blood work, it may be his last. You're at your wits' end trying to select the perfect present. A one-year subscription to *Entertainment Weekly* might be overly optimistic. Somehow a case of Sustecal lacks that personal touch. Why not consider a LifeStyle Urn™?

Yes, in that vast suburban mall known as Amerika, Land of the Free (to Shop Till You Drop) and Home of the Grave, an innovative company called LifeStyle Urns™ has started marketing cremation urns designed specifically for the gay community. One urn has a lambda carved on the top panel, symbolizing gay pride. Another has a rosebud, symbolizing peace; a third is gracefully smooth on all sides. And, yes, there is a twenty-four-hour toll-free number (1-800-685-URNS) for catalog and order information. The press release (accompanied by a refrigerator magnet and a Rolodex card) states: "By offering the privacy of at-home catalog shopping, LifeStyle Urns™ serves those who are ill with AIDS."

I for one associate the term "lifestyle" with condoms and

Originally appeared as "Urn Your Keep" in Out, *December/January 1994.*

Robin Leach. But I guess that "DeathStyle" would be too morbid. I'm sure it's only a matter of time before Ivana Trump starts hawking LifeStyle Urns™ on the Home Shopping Network. One day you'll be walking through your favorite department store and hear the loudspeakers boom: "Attention, Kmart shoppers! We have a blue-light special in aisle thirty! Fifty percent off on Life-Style Urns™ for the next fifteen minutes."

Last Sunday I called them up for further information.

"Hello. Is this LifeStyle Urns™? Could you tell me how much your cremation urns go for? . . .

"Gee, that's pretty expensive. Do you ever have sales? Do you sell seconds at a warehouse outlet? Like maybe when you were doing sample runs, you did a few with the lambda on backward? . . .

"You don't? You see, my lover, Bernard, just died last week and the problem is the insurance barely paid for the memorial service. I'm kind of low on funds myself, since I had to quit my job and go on public assistance last fall. It looks like I'll be a goner in a couple of months, too, so I really don't see why I need an urn for the mantelpiece that will last forever. His family disowned him when they found out he was gay. Most of his friends are already dead. Do you have any slightly damaged urns? Ones that biodegrade in a few years? Do you have any urns that are cracked on the bottom, so nobody would know?"

But of course I didn't actually call them.

I was too appalled.

Is this crass commercialism? Is this tasteless exploitation? Or is it just another example of niche marketing in our consumer marketplace?

I admit I had my doubts about this product until I read the tag line on the press release:

"LifeStyle Urns™: The Dignified Choice."

Regrets

I've never been to Greece.

I waited until I was nineteen to have sex.

I had sex with the wrong person in 1982.

I had anal sex with the wrong person in 1982.

I had anal sex without a condom with the wrong person in 1982.

I had anal sex without a condom with the wrong person in 1982 and got infected with HIV.

I had anal sex without a condom with the wrong person in 1982 and got infected with HIV and warts.

I went to Gluteus Maximus, M.D., and suffered the consequences.

I allowed someone to slip his dick into my asshole and fuck me without a condom in 1984 even though he tricked me into it, but especially because he said he couldn't possibly be positive because he was only a top.

I didn't have wild sex with drugs in 1979 because I was too shy, restrained, conservative, neurotic, and a mess besides; I was afraid of chemicals and the addictive personality. I never really binged and purged and went crazy and drank excessively and didn't suffer the next day. I did drugs only a few times (I wonder if heroin would have been nice), and the only solace is that I may end up trying morphine at the end.

I believe that there may be some possibility of transmitting HIV infection through oral sex, and consequently, my HIV-negative boyfriends of the past haven't been able to blow me on a regular basis.

I didn't try water sports even though my boyfriend was rather insistent.

I never got used to anal intercourse.

I never rimmed anyone in 1979.

I never rimmed anyone without Saran Wrap, period.

I never jerked off Vito in the Chelsea Gym steam room.

I never was fist-fucked.

I never really let go.

I never found my G spot.

I never made it with a lesbian.

I had sex with a former health-care professional of mine in his office.

I had sex with a former health-care professional of mine in his office during an appointment.

I had sex with a former health-care professional of mine in his office during an appointment when there were several people in the waiting room.

I had sex with a former health-care professional of mine in his office during an appointment when there were several people in the waiting room, and he charged for the entire session.

When I found out that Harold was dating Barry, for whom I lusted and would never have again, I spent an hour regaling Harold with rude and sordid tales about his therapist that were unfortunately true.

I didn't get arrested at the Supreme Court in 1988 to protest the *Hardwick* decision.

I never found religion.

I don't believe in an afterlife.

I don't believe there is anything after death.

I never paid proper attention to astrology.

I didn't charge more things on Visa before declaring bankruptcy.

I didn't move out of that hellhole in Hell's Kitchenette for thirteen years.

I was such a snob that in college I didn't major in applied mathematics, I majored in pure.

I didn't go to that interview for a mathematician at the jet-propulsion lab because I had already accepted a job as a computer programmer.

I'm still at my fucking job at the Modern Language Association after twelve years and counting.

I wasn't attracted enough to John to be his boyfriend.

I didn't fall in love with Mark.

I didn't follow Daniel to Minneapolis.

I allowed my fear of insanity and change and strangeness to get in the way of possible relationships with promising people.

My worst nightmare came true when I realized I not only had become my mother, but I married her.

I never really fell in love, only lust.

I never got in touch with my feelings.

I never admitted I had feelings.

I didn't call home enough.

I didn't speak with my mother every other week.

I didn't speak with my sister every other week.

I didn't diligently visit my grandmother after she lost her mind.

I didn't save any of my father's boring letters that he wrote to me when I was a freshman in college, and he died when I was a sophomore.

I was never able to completely turn off the voice in my head I call "Mother." No matter what I do or say, this voice always has a prompt rejoinder. It is rarely pleasant, useful, or appropriate to the situation.

I've hurt people intentionally and unintentionally with my writing.

I never found the proper therapist, editor, or agent.

I would have sold out and written a television situation comedy for half a piece of silver, but nobody offered.

I didn't write every day.

I didn't floss enough.

I never stopped biting my nails or picking my nose.

I didn't try to file down the warts on my hands with a pumice stone every night until my palms bled.

I always hid in the bathroom when strange men came over to the apartment to fix things.

I never was assertive with salespeople.

I never learned how to make small talk to the person who was cutting my hair.

I am too shallow for words.

I was duplicitous and complained about all my friends behind their backs to my other friends.

I allowed my life to be ruled by guilt and regrets.

I allowed my life to be ruled by questionnaires found in *Ladies' Home Journal, Family Circle,* and *Cosmopolitan.*

I never lived in Europe.

I never hitchhiked across the country.

I didn't become a full-time AIDS treatment activist.

I didn't do anything substantive to end the AIDS crisis except whine at an unnaturally high pitch.

I didn't go to the Montreal International AIDS Conference even though I was invited.

I didn't go to the Cultural Festival in Vancouver coinciding with the Gay Games because I didn't respond "yes" for a month and by then it was too late.

I made an utter fool of myself at the New York Public Library with John Weir.

I have held grudges for more than ten years.

I have thought ill of the dead.

I have said inappropriate things in a loud voice at memorial services.

I'm not going to see the coming of the new millennium.

I never had a half share on the Island.

A lot of people say they've lived their lives with no regrets. They're lying.

The
Last
Piece

I could continue in this vein indefinitely. Future episodes could include: Davey gets a cane. Davey gets a Hickman catheter and matching bag and shoes. Davey goes blind. Davey loses all control of his limbs. Davey goes on total parenteral nutrition. Davey gets a walker. Davey gets his oxygen tube entangled with the telephone wire. Davey complains about not being able to wear a simple shift over the catheter and tubes. Davey develops Tourette's syndrome. Davey finds religion. Davey becomes even more bitter than before.

But there comes a point when your sense of humor grows stale. It's time for a break. Writing these essays becomes too much of a strain. I've lost my taste for it. I can only mask so much bitterness and anger with humor. The subject ceases to be palatable. It all gets too ugly.

I'm beginning to lose perspective. I need more distance. I cannot write about being ill when I am ill. Now I wonder more and more: Should I quit my job after my first opportunistic infection? Should I quit it after my second? Should I not even wait that long and hope my finances and health insurance hold up?

I have the sneaking suspicion that circumstances will determine the outcome and any conscious decision I make will be moot.

We can leave here with the hopeful fiction that nothing worse will happen, that the cure is just around the corner, but that would be fooling no one, least of all myself.

I could look back from the perspective of beyond the plague.

I can't.

This is the logical stopping place.

I want to forget everything I've been through, everything my brave friends have gone through, dead and alive.

I want to pretend that none of this is happening.

I want to go into denial and never resurface.

I'm tired of AIDS.

Most days I find two AIDS obituaries in *The New York Times*.

Last July, after Tim Bailey's aborted political funeral, I became profoundly depressed. The world was shrouded in the heavy fog of death. Each step I took made me feel as though I were submerged in black water. The sadness was unbearable.

Life was a meaningless cycle: work, sleep, work, sleep, work, sleep, work, sleep, with the occasional vacation to break up the monotony. I check off items from my ridiculously inane to-do list. I make new lists. What's the point? Why bother going on?

Does writing actually help anything?

People die every day. Eventually I will die.

I'm afraid of what the next year will bring.

I'm exhausted.

I don't want to think about it anymore.

I fear I am repeating myself.

So this is the end, for now, of my *Trilogy of Terror.* Thank you for indulging me in my personal *Portrait of the Artist as a Young Diseased Jew Fag Pariah.* Thank you for listening to *The Absolutely True*

Confessions of a Guilty AIDS Victim. This *Briefing for a Descent into Hell* has been brought to you by many corporate sponsor, including Burroughs Wellcome, Hoffmann–La Roche, Jenruction, LifeStyle Urns™, and the Chubb Medical Group. Special thanks go to Senator Jesse Helms, John Cardinal O'Conn former Representative William Dannemeyer, and the religio Right for their efforts in prolonging the epidemic. This conclude our presentation of *Chronicles of a Death Foretold.* Good-bye, and good luck.

Confessions of a Guilty AIDS Victim. This *Briefing for a Descent into Hell* has been brought to you by many corporate sponsors, including Burroughs Wellcome, Hoffmann–La Roche, Hemasuction, LifeStyle Urns™, and the Chubb Medical Group. Special thanks go to Senator Jesse Helms, John Cardinal O'Connor, former Representative William Dannemeyer, and the religious Right for their efforts in prolonging the epidemic. This concludes our presentation of *Chronicles of a Death Foretold.* Good-bye, and good luck.

FOR THE BEST IN PAPERBACKS, LOOK FOR THE

In every corner of the world, on every subject under the sun, Penguin represents quality and variety—the very best in publishing today.

For complete information about books available from Penguin—including Puffins, Penguin Classics, and Arkana—and how to order them, write to us at the appropriate address below. Please note that for copyright reasons the selection of books varies from country to country.

In the United Kingdom: Please write to *Dept. JC, Penguin Books Ltd, FREEPOST, West Drayton, Middlesex UB7 0BR.*

If you have any difficulty in obtaining a title, please send your order with the correct money, plus ten percent for postage and packaging, to *P.O. Box No. 11, West Drayton, Middlesex UB7 0BR*

In the United States: Please write to *Consumer Sales, Penguin USA, P.O. Box 999, Dept. 17109, Bergenfield, New Jersey 07621-0120.* VISA and MasterCard holders call 1-800-253-6476 to order all Penguin titles

In Canada: Please write to *Penguin Books Canada Ltd, 10 Alcorn Avenue, Suite 300, Toronto, Ontario M4V 3B2*

In Australia: Please write to *Penguin Books Australia Ltd, P.O. Box 257, Ringwood, Victoria 3134*

In New Zealand: Please write to *Penguin Books (NZ) Ltd, Private Bag 102902, North Shore Mail Centre, Auckland 10*

In India: Please write to *Penguin Books India Pvt Ltd, 706 Eros Apartments, 56 Nehru Place, New Delhi 110 019*

In the Netherlands: Please write to *Penguin Books Netherlands bv, Postbus 3507, NL-1001 AH Amsterdam*

In Germany: Please write to *Penguin Books Deutschland GmbH, Metzlerstrasse 26, 60594 Frankfurt am Main*

In Spain: Please write to *Penguin Books S. A., Bravo Murillo 19, 1° B, 28015 Madrid*

In Italy: Please write to *Penguin Italia s.r.l., Via Felice Casati 20, I-20124 Milano*

In France: Please write to *Penguin France S. A., 17 rue Lejeune, F–31000 Toulouse*

In Japan: Please write to *Penguin Books Japan, Ishikiribashi Building, 2–5–4, Suido, Bunkyo-ku, Tokyo 112*

In Greece: Please write to *Penguin Hellas Ltd, Dimocritou 3, GR–106 71 Athens*

In South Africa: Please write to *Longman Penguin Southern Africa (Pty) Ltd, Private Bag X08, Bertsham 2013.*